COLOUR GUI

Forensic pathology

David J. Williams BSc(Hons) MB ChB MSc PhD MRC Path
  DMJ(Path) FRCPA
Specialist Forensic Pathologist, John Tonge Centre for Forensic Sciences
Clinical Associate Professor, Department of Pathology, University of Queensland,
  Australia

Anthony J. Ansford MB ChB DCP(Otago) FRACP FRCPA
Director, John Tonge Centre for Forensic Sciences
Adjunct Professor, Faculty of Science & Technology, Griffith University
Clinical Associate Professor, Department of Pathology, University of Queensland,
  Australia

David S. Priday Dip MT MAIMS
Supervising Scientist, Forensic Pathology, John Tonge Centre for Forensic Sciences,
  Australia

Alex S. Forrest BDSc Grad Cert Ed
Consultant Forensic Odontologist, John Tonge Centre for Forensic Sciences,
  Australia

CHURCHILL
LIVINGSTONE

EDINBURGH LONDON NEW YORK PHILADELPHIA
SYDNEY TORONTO 1998

CHURCHILL LIVINGSTONE
An imprint of Harcourt Brace and Company Limited

© Pearson Professional Limited 1996
© Harcourt Brace and Company Limited 1998

⬭ is a registered trademark of Harcourt Brace and
Company Limited

First published 1996
  Reprinted 1998

ISBN 0 443 05388 X

British Library Cataloguing in Publication Data
A catalogue record for this book is available from the
British Library

Library of Congress Cataloging in Publication Data
A catalog record for this book is available from the
Library of Congress

Medical knowledge is constantly changing. As new information
becomes available, changes in treatment, procedures,
equipment and the use of drugs become necessary. The authors
and the publishers have, as far as it is possible, taken care to
ensure that the information given in this text is accurate and up
to date. However, readers are strongly advised to confirm the
information, especially with regard to drug usage, complies with
current legislation and standards of practice.

Publisher
Timothy Horne
Project Editor
Jim Killgore
Production
Kay Hunston
Design Direction
Erik Bigland

The
publisher's
policy is to use
**paper manufactured
from sustainable forests**

Produced by Addison Wesley Longman China Limited, Hong Kong
WW/02

Preface

This volume in the Colour Guide series provides brief notes and colour illustrations on selected aspects of forensic pathology. It is not intended as a comprehensive coverage of the topic but rather to highlight some general principles and examine some grey areas. It is anticipated that the book will be of value to medical students and also to those practitioners who may be called upon from time to time to perform forensic autopsies. It will also prove useful to students and practitioners in the legal profession including coroners and barristers practising in criminal law.

It is tempting in the preparation of a book of this type to use the best available photographs. We have tried to select photographs on their practical value rather than their aesthetic appeal, however. We feel that this approach may be of very real assistance to medical practitioners performing autopsies under difficult circumstances.

John Tonge Centre
Brisbane
1996

DJW
AJA
DSP
ASF

Acknowledgments

Mrs Sandie Brighton and Mrs Di Keller are thanked for preparation of the text. Mr Jim O'Sullivan, Commissioner of Police, Queensland Police Service, is thanked for permission to use certain police photographs. The publishers of The Courier-Mail are thanked for permission to use one of their photographs. Pathologists from Brisbane are thanked for their assistance, particularly Richard Steele, Charles Naylor, Tony Tannenberg and Di Cominos.

The staff of Queensland Health Scientific Services are appreciated for their assistance, particularly Michele Sullivan, Bronwyn Parker and Kevin Chalmers. Contributions from Professor R. M. N. MacSween, Professor M. Moore, Dr Melissa Elkins, Dr L. Walsh and Dr Caroline Acton are also appreciated.

Contents

1 / Introduction to forensic pathology

Definition Pathology is the study of disease and tissue injury by scientific methods. Forensic pathology is a specialized branch of pathology which relates to the effects of trauma, poisoning, occupational hazards and natural disease within a legal framework. The forensic pathologist would usually perform an autopsy or post-mortem examination on the instruction or order of a legal authority and such an examination is directed towards the public good.

The purpose of a post-mortem examination goes far beyond determining the cause of death. The investigation of the relative contributions to the death of trauma and natural disease are of particular importance. Reconstruction of the events surrounding the death is one of the prime achievements of the investigation.

Benefits to the community from the work of the forensic pathologist include:

- identification of disease patterns
- notification of infectious agents
- the detection of homicide and of foul play
- identification of mutilated, decomposed or incinerated human remains.

The last point is important in that identification of the deceased may allow the relatives to complete their grief process.

Safety The performance of post-mortem examinations is a potentially hazardous process and stringent health and safety procedures apply. Simple safeguards, such as cut-proof gloves (Fig. 1) worn under the surgical gloves, are routinely employed and, for dangerous cases, more complex safety equipment may be used.

In modern mortuaries, there is often a division into 'clean' and 'dirty' areas. The pathologist changes into surgical scrub gear and rubber boots before venturing into the dirty area, where the post-mortem examination takes place. Photography and video recording are commonly used to document the findings in controversial cases.

The audience for the post-mortem examination, be they police officers, medical students or other medical practitioners, can view the findings from behind glass (Fig. 2), while sitting comfortably in the clean area.

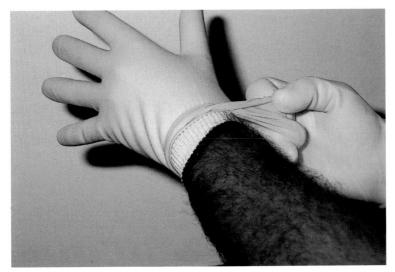

Fig. 1 Cut-proof glove.

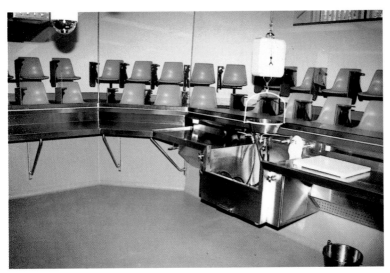

Fig. 2 Autopsy demonstration area.

2 / **The death scene**

The police may require medical attendance at the scene of a death. Such attendance is a useful exercise in that valuable police time may be saved if the death turns out to be non-suspicious. In suspicious cases, observations made at the scene may help explain certain of the post-mortem examination findings.

Equipment Forensic pathologists attending such scenes frequently may carry:

1. *A 'murder bag'.* This contains a collection of useful equipment relevant to the examination of a corpse. A thermometer can be used to determine the temperature of the corpse and the ambient temperature of the surroundings.
2. *A camera.* A polaroid camera provides an immediate photographic record of the scene.
3. *Protective clothing.* Scenes are often extremely unpleasant; protective overalls, gloves and rubber boots are recommended. The attending pathologist must ensure that he does not contribute any trace evidence to the scene.
4. *Torch and map.* The police may provide adequate lighting at the scene but a torch is a useful back-up. The torch is also useful for studying the map and also road signs on the way to the scene.
5. *Notepad and pen or portable tape recorder* to record information, sketches and other observations.

The illustrations demonstrate two cases where a visit to the scene was worthwhile. In one (Fig. 3), a young girl was found on a building site with severe head injuries and her skirt hitched up. The proximity of the building blocks and the abrasions of her feet made sexual attack unlikely. Examination of the site showed a steel beam bearing her footprints (Fig. 4). She had fallen while intoxicated. In the other case, a suicidal hanging (Fig. 5) went badly wrong, although it was still fatal. The position of the rope explained the abrasions behind the knee and the extensive facial abrasions (Fig. 6).

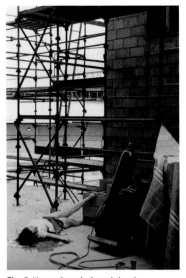

Fig. 3 Young female found dead.

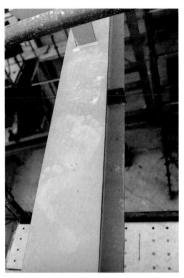

Fig. 4 The footprints of the deceased.

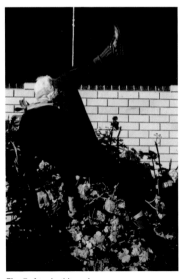

Fig. 5 Atypical hanging.

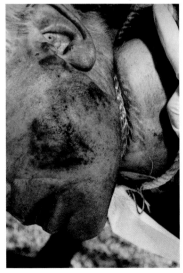

Fig. 6 Facial abrasions in hanging.

Investigations ***Important questions relevant to the death scene***

- If the deceased was found in a property, was that property secure?
- Has the body been moved since death?
- Has the property been ransacked?
- Is the death a disguised homicide?
- If a weapon has been used, is that weapon with the body?
- Is there sexual interference?
- In a suspected gunshot suicide, are there any textbooks of anatomy, demonstrating vital organs, at the scene?
- Is there potential danger to investigators at the scene, for example a live electrical conductor?
- Is there any evidence of self-mutilation or drug abuse?

The important question as to whether the death is due to natural causes, accident, suicide or homicide may have to be deferred until the post-mortem examination is performed.

Infrequently, an unusual suicide may result from ideas stimulated by the media. 1 week after a film depicting a lawn mower going berserk inside a house, an elderly man was found dead with his motorized lawn mower in the bedroom. He had died of carbon monoxide poisoning. He had presumably removed his hearing aids (Fig. 7) so that the noise of the lawn mower was eliminated.

The use of pulleys and levers as an aid to suicide is not infrequent. In Figure 8, residual string from a simple pulley system involving a log is seen around the trigger of the rifle.

The scene in Figure 9 looks at first glance to suggest homicide. The body has numerous puncture wounds, resembling stab wounds. The creek, however, is full of crocodiles and the deceased had tried to swim across.

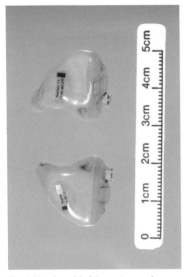

Fig. 7 Hearing aids (clues at scene).

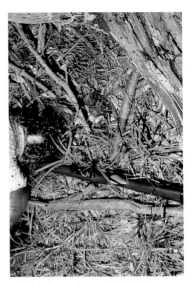

Fig. 8 String and log arrangement.

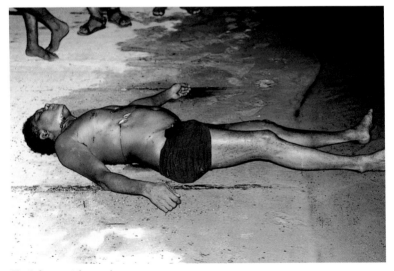

Fig. 9 Scene at the creek.

3 / **Time of death**

Cooling

Corpses, in general, cool progressively after death and there has been much scientific investigation into assessing methods for measuring post-mortem interval.

Homeostasis 'Normal' body temperature is subject to individual variation, circadian rhythm, emotional stress, disease states, metabolic problems, circulatory disturbances, drug effects.

Factors Heat loss from a corpse is dependent upon:

1. physical size
2. insulation
3. body support
4. environmental factors.

Clothing and fat act as effective insulation while a large body has a greater surface area from which to lose heat. Water immersion cools a body much more quickly than does exposure to the air. Moving air is more conducive to cooling the body than stagnant air. Cold surfaces, for example the floor of a deep freeze, are obviously much more effective at cooling the body than a hot surface, such as lying on an electric blanket.

The putrefied body

Sources of information In cases where there is advanced putrefaction or skeletonization, observation of such mundane items as bus tickets, milk cartons, cheque book stubs and so on may reveal useful information as to the approximate time of death. Identification of insect predators (entomology) and physicochemical tests on bones may also yield important information. Entomology is one of the more useful methods of assessing time period since death in putrefied bodies.

The appearance of putrefaction itself (Fig. 10) is a poor guide to the time that has elapsed since death. Blowfly larvae (Fig. 11) examination is much more valuable. A knowledge of botany is occasionally useful in cases of bodies buried in a garden (Fig. 12), where there may be interference with the rooting systems of large shrubs. The skull had been buried for 5 years.

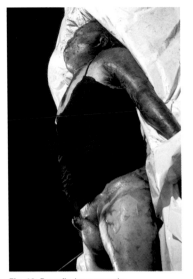

Fig. 10 Putrefied transvestite.

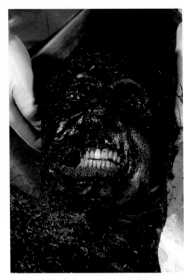

Fig. 11 Blowfly larvae on putrefying Caucasian.

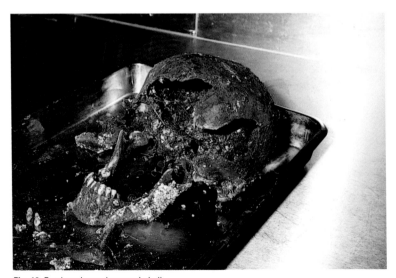

Fig. 12 Retrieved axe-damaged skull.

4 / Post-mortem changes

Rigor mortis

Features
Rigor mortis describes the stiffening of muscles as ATP breaks down after death. The development of rigor has tremendous variation and may be hastened by certain poisons or by certain types of death, such as electrocution.

Rigor is preceded by a primary flaccidity and is followed by secondary flaccidity.

If a body is found in an illogical posture, that is, a posture which would not have been maintained during primary flaccidity, it implies that the body has been moved during rigor.

Rigor may render the examination of certain parts of the body, for example the palmar aspects of the hands, difficult. Crucial lesions, such as electrical burns or defence injuries, may be missed if the rigor is not overcome.

Putrefaction

Features
Putrefactive changes in the tissues render visual identification difficult and may mask or mimic trauma or natural disease. Figure 13 shows an example of putrefied hypertrophic obstructive cardiomyopathy (HOCM). Putrefactive bacteria, commonly clostridia, break down the components of the blood to form a frothy, greasy mix. Froth in the heart in a putrefied body must not be diagnosed as air embolism; the gas formation is also a common cause of dilated chambers.

One of the earliest features of putrefaction is a greenish discoloration to the abdomen. Spread of putrefactive bacteria in the blood may produce haemolysis, such that peripheral blood vessels demonstrate a green-purple arborescent pattern known as marbling (Fig. 14). Bodies in the water tend not to show such florid colour changes, especially if the blood is leached out by sea water (Fig. 15).

A major problem caused by putrefaction is the production of artefacts. The breakdown of proteins can produce amines and other substances which may be mistaken for drugs.

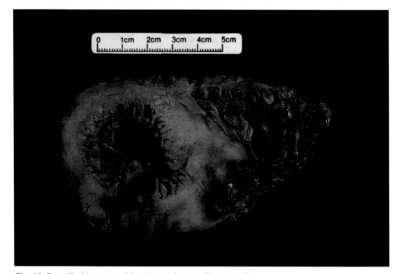

Fig. 13 Putrefied hypertrophic obstructive cardiomyopathy.

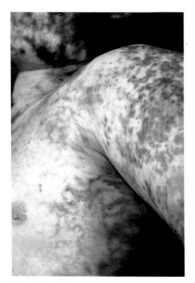

Fig. 14 Marbling and putrefactive blotchiness.

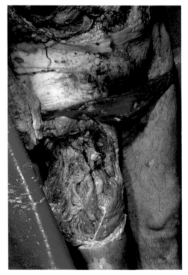

Fig. 15 Shark bite and putrefaction (in sea water).

Hypostasis

Features   Hypostasis describes the gravitational movement of blood into the lower parts of the body and its individual organs after death. The blood remains within the vascular system.

The timing of hypostasis and of any subsequent coagulation is variable.

The importance of hypostasis is that if found in an inappropriate distribution relative to the body position, then movement of the body is implied.

For a body found in the supine position, hypostasis is normally diffusely spread over the back except for areas of contact with the supporting surface (usually shoulders, buttocks and calves). Coarse or blotchy blue-red spots occurring in an area of hypostasis should not be confused with the fine petechiae of asphyxia. Hypostasis is frequently patterned. A naked body lying on a tiled floor, for example, may demonstrate a pattern of hypostasis corresponding to the gaps between the tiles (Figs 16 & 17).

Colour   The normal colour of hypostasis is bluish-red. Different colours may be encountered as a result of poisoning, disease or environmental factors.

Pink hypostasis. Pink hypostasis is classically seen in carbon monoxide poisoning but it is also a feature of cyanide poisoning, hypothermia, refrigeration and aerosol inhalation (Fig. 18).

Internal hypostasis

Hypostatic engorgement in the lower parts of the lung may be mistaken for pneumonia. Similarly, hypostasis in the heart can be confused with infarction. These problems are solved by histological examination.

Putrefaction and hypostasis

In the supine body, there may be incomplete emptying of the superficial veins because of functioning valves in the veins draining the head. This phenomenon leaves small pockets of hypostasis, which may mimic areas of bruising, particularly when putrefaction supervenes.

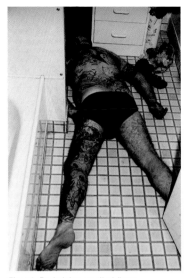

Fig. 16 Body lying on tiled floor.

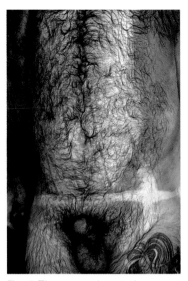

Fig. 17 Tile pattern to hypostasis.

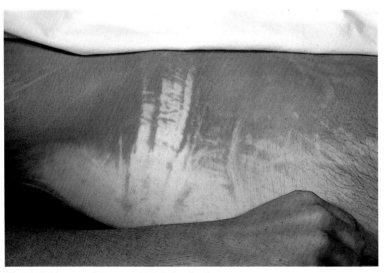

Fig. 18 Pink hypostasis in aerosol inhalation death.

5 / **Identification**

Value The correct identification of a body or body fragment is of major medico-legal importance. This identification is based on scrutiny of innate physical characteristics shown by the body and also on inspection of acquired characteristics.

Innate characteristics The innate physical characteristics include such features as:

- facial appearance
- body build and stature, including skeletal structure
- skin pigmentation
- hair and eye colour
- tooth and hair structure
- fingerprints
- race
- biological indices, such as blood group serology, DNA profile and secretor status.

Certain of these characteristics may be altered significantly by post-mortem changes. Putrefaction, for example, may cause the iris of the eye to darken, the hair to fall out and the soft tissues to become bloated and discoloured.

Acquired characteristics Acquired characteristics include:

- occupational stigmata
- scars (Fig. 19)
- brands (Fig. 20)
- tattoos (Fig. 21)
- clothing and personal effects
- jewellery (Fig. 21)
- disease
- dental repairs
- prosthetic devices (Fig. 22).

Fingerprints, clothing, the contents of a wallet or handbag and other personal effects are regularly used to confirm a tentative visual identification of the body. When there is some degree of mutilation or putrefaction, it is usual not to have visual identification but to rely on these confirmatory techniques supplemented perhaps by foot, palm and lips prints and also by dental identification.

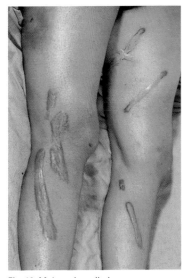

Fig. 19 Melanesian tribal scars.

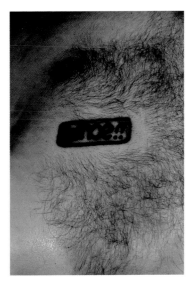

Fig. 20 Brand mark.

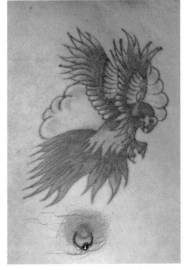

Fig. 21 Tattoo and silver nipple ring.

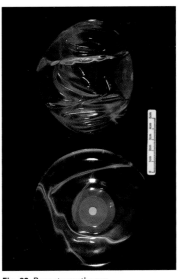

Fig. 22 Breast prostheses.

Skeletal remains   The identification of skeletal remains presents special problems and the pertinent questions to ask are:

- Are the bones human?
- How many individuals?
- Can the primary characteristics of the deceased, that is, sex, race, age and height, be established?
- Has the death occurred within the past 50 years?

X-ray studies are particularly useful for the investigation of features such as disease patterns, shape of sinuses, occurrence of prosthetic devices, fractures and asymmetry of paired bones. Such features as the trabecular pattern of normal bones may be a crucial factor in identification.

Post-mortem radiographs are compared with radiographs retrieved from the medical records of a suspected deceased (Fig. 23).

Dental identification   Dentures and other prosthetic devices are sometimes clearly marked as to where they were made and by whom. A patient's record number is also a possible finding.

In other cases, dental identification comprises comparison of dental charts of the presumed deceased with the post-mortem remains. Ideally, the jaws are removed to facilitate examination (Fig. 24).

Possible outcomes of the process include:

- identity established (Fig. 25)
- identity consistent with but not established beyond doubt
- insufficient data for a valid comparison
- identity definitely not established.

Problems that may be encountered include:

- incorrect tooth identification, either ante-mortem or post-mortem
- incorrect charting by ante-mortem dentist
- inadequate documentation of procedures by ante-mortem dentist
- inadequate ante-mortem radiographs
- difficulties in interpretation of ante-mortem records
- incomplete ante-mortem records.

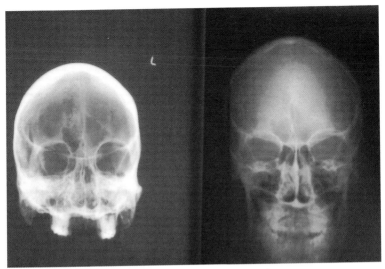

Fig. 23 Comparison of ante-mortem and post-mortem radiographs.

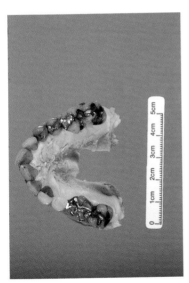

Fig. 24 Upper jaw removed.

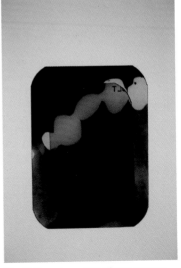

Fig. 25 Superimposition of ante-mortem and post-mortem radiographs of dental bridge.

Facial reproduction This technique is an anatomical exercise based on employing a database to characterize usual soft tissue thicknesses at a multitude of points on the normal skull. It is important to know certain primary characteristics of the deceased, particularly race and sex, before attempting facial reproduction.

In the absence of any other leads to identity, forensic facial reproduction may be employed to create a likeness of the face from cranial remains. Soft tissues are modelled on the bony remains either by hand or by sophisticated computer graphic techniques. The technique is more useful for adolescent and adult persons than it is for children.

The reconstruction is not intended for use as proof of identity. The main value of the reconstruction is that it can be displayed to public scrutiny in an effort to establish leads to identification.

In our experience, computer imaging provides a very rapid method for successful application of the technique. The cranial remains are available for examination throughout the exercise. An audit trail of stages is kept and can be displayed on demand. Alterations can be made in the light of new information quickly and easily, without changing previous images. Monochrome imaging of the reconstruction avoids the need for concern about complexion and eye colour which are likely to be unknown, and provides the best response from the public. In the technique we favour, the resulting images are designed to be midway between an artistic rendition and photo-realism (Figs 26, 27 & 28).

The face shown in Figure 28 is purely a theoretical image. The two sides of the face demonstrate how the computer imaging can be altered to suggest a particular age.

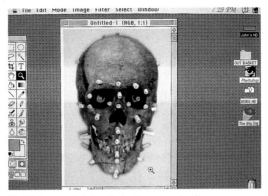

Fig. 26 Image of skull with depth markers in situ.

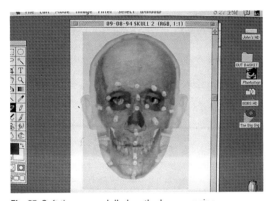

Fig. 27 Soft tissues modelled on the bony remains.

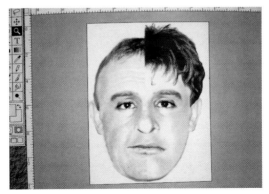

Fig. 28 Theoretical image.

Photographic
superimposition

Photographic superimposition is a technique used to compare the facial features of the alleged deceased and the cranial remains. It relies on the same database of soft tissue thicknesses as does facial reproduction. The post-mortem image is captured with particular attention being paid to matching the camera angle and camera–subject distance of the ante-mortem photograph to avoid perspective errors. The two images are then superimposed, and tissue thicknesses examined (Fig. 29).

This process has been facilitated by the use of video cameras such that two images, one of the photograph and the other of the skull, are mixed on one video display unit. More recently, digital image manipulation techniques have provided significant advantages over previous methods. These include the ability to take the computer into court and demonstrate the technique before a judge and jury. An audit trail of the various steps involved can be kept for validation.

A variation on this technique is the application of image superimposition of the dentition to questions of identification. In cases where sufficient anterior teeth remain on the cranium, and a photograph is available which shows the suspected deceased smiling, superimposition of the upper anterior teeth can be sufficient to establish identity beyond doubt. In cases when colour ante-mortem photographs are available, colour imaging should be used, since various colours of the teeth and restorations can contribute a great deal to the effectiveness of the result.

Figures 30 and 31 show a case in which the identity of the deceased was established solely on the basis of such a comparison. The image quality is poor as a result of the very small size of the original ante-mortem photograph, but the upper anterior dentition of the deceased was sufficiently distinctive for there to be no doubt as to the validity of the comparison. It is important to resist the temptation to use digital image editing techniques to 'improve' the quality of images such as these. The ability to perform the comparison in real time before a jury more than compensates for the poor image quality.

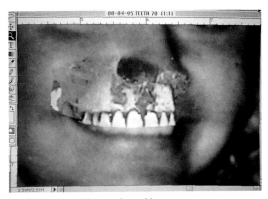

Fig. 29 Photographic superimposition.

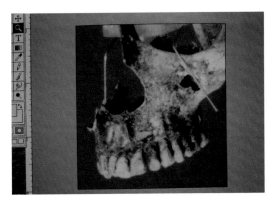

Fig. 30 Upper jaw and maxilla.

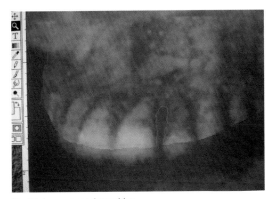

Fig. 31 Image superimposition.

6 / External appearances

Certain external appearances of a body may generate alarm or suspicion and it is important for the forensic pathologist to exclude homicide. Common conditions which regularly produce contentious cases include:

Alcoholism The complications of alcohol abuse are numerous but the tendency to fall over, the occurrence of epileptic fits and the presence of liver damage, with the attendant problem of poor blood clotting, are frequent innocent explanations for a body being found in a suspicious condition (Fig. 32).

Alcoholics are, of course, frequently involved in violent confrontations. The story, the appearance at the scene, and the autopsy with toxicological studies, are usually sufficient to explain the events that led to the death.

Infection Infection can cause death very quickly, even in the healthiest individual, and may produce diverse external appearances in doing so. Infection combined with disseminated intravascular coagulation (DIC) sometimes causes blotchy purplish, red or pink rashes which may be mistaken for bruises or abrasions (Fig. 33). The converse is also true, in that bruises may be misdiagnosed as the Waterhouse–Friderichsen syndrome.

Infection in just one organ, especially a genital organ, may be misdiagnosed as violence to that organ.

Figure 34 demonstrates a late complication of lighting a firework embedded in the anus.

Haematological abnormalities Haemorrhage is the loss of blood from the circulation, usually due to trauma. A tendency to spontaneous and excessive bleeding is termed a haemorrhagic diathesis. Such a diathesis may cause problems in the estimation of the force required to produce various wounds and haematomas. Assessment of any bony damage associated with the injury may provide more reliable information.

Surgery It is not uncommon for a deceased to have surgery prior to death and the surgical intervention may occasionally cause problems in the interpretation of wounds. Discussions with the surgeon or even asking him or her to attend the autopsy should clarify matters.

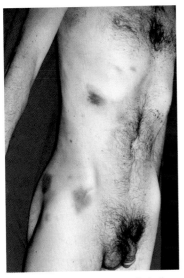

Fig. 32 Multiple bruises on an alcoholic.

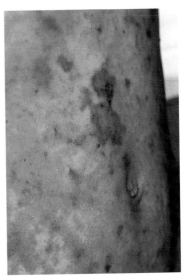

Fig. 33 Blotchy rash in disseminated intravascular coagulation.

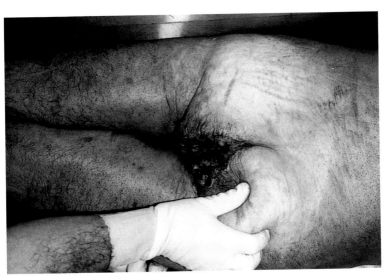

Fig. 34 Anal gangrene.

7 / Wounds

Definition   There are legal definitions of a wound in certain countries but, for practical purposes, a wound is traumatic damage to any part of the body.

Classification   Wounds are classified according to their appearance and there are four main types.

Bruise. When blood vessels are damaged by mechanical impact, a bruise may result. A fresh bruise in the skin is seen as a purple or red-black area. A bruise will change colour as time passes (Fig. 35) but estimation of a time interval when assessing a particular bruise is unreliable. It is commonly more valid to state that certain bruises are of different ages.

A bruise within an organ is more commonly described as a contusion.

Periorbital bruising is popularly known as 'a black eye'. Such an injury may follow the direct application of force to the eye or may be consequent to the gravitational movement of blood either from an injured forehead or from a fracture of the base of the skull.

Bruises inflicted just prior to death may not be seen at autopsy but may appear some days after the autopsy.

Abrasion. An abrasion is an area of grazing of the skin, caused by the tangential impact of a roughened surface (Fig. 36). Ante-mortem abrasions are typically red-brown when fresh and they may dry out to produce a glazed, brown parchment-like appearance.

In common with bruises, abrasions may demonstrate a pattern, depending on the nature of the applied force.

Laceration. This is a full thickness tear or split in the skin (Fig. 37). A laceration inflicted on skin which overlies bone may mimic an incised wound to the uninitiated. A laceration tends to have crushed margins with tissue bridges and associated abrasion and bruising. The term can also be used to describe a tear in an internal organ.

Incised wound. An incised wound is a cut produced by a sharp instrument such as a knife or piece of glass (Fig. 38). There are two common variants of the incised wound, a slash and a stab wound. A slash is a cut of greater length than depth. A stab wound is a penetrating injury where the depth of penetration is greater than the surface length of the wound.

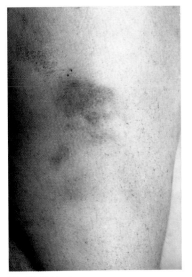

Fig. 35 Old bruise.

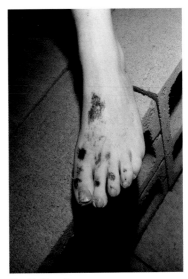

Fig. 36 Abrasions.

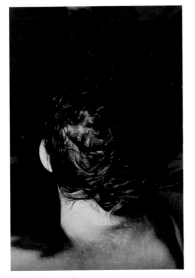

Fig. 37 Laceration.

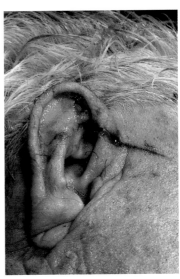

Fig. 38 Incised wound caused by glass.

8 / Patterned injuries

Electrocution

Domestic electricity

A shock occurs when a person is not insulated from the passage of electricity. The fatal passage of electricity may cause entry and exit wounds, sometimes of a patterned nature, but they may be absent if there is a broad area of contact. Electrical burns (Joule burns) present as intact or collapsed blisters, keratin nodules or skin pits (Fig. 39). Typically there is an areola of blackened skin around the pale contact mark, but there may be a rim of erythema around a blackened centre (Fig. 40).

Entry burns are usually more severe than exit burns and they may demonstrate a distinct colour due to metallization from the conductor.

It is important to thoroughly clean the hands and to overcome the effects of rigor when examining the hands, as the appearance of an electrical burn may be very subtle. Similarly, if there is a history of an electrical contact to the head, it may be necessary to shave an area of head hair.

Accidental electrocution is occasionally diagnosed only at post-mortem examination and a priority then is to prevent a repetition of the accident. In suicidal electrocution, the apparatus and wires are found in situ and there may be very prominent metallization of the electrocuted skin.

High-voltage electricity

High-voltage electrical cables commonly occur near railway lines and may be touched accidentally. The high voltage can propel the body some distance and causes charring of the skin, typically with a 'crocodile-skin' appearance which may also be seen in lightning fatalities (Fig. 41).

Lightning

Torn and scorched clothing may be noted on the body. Metallic objects may show a welded appearance (Fig. 42) or demonstrate magnetism. Infrequently, a fern-like pattern of skin mottling (arborescent markings) is seen. In lightning strike, there is not only a very high voltage but there is a blast wave produced by the discharge of electricity through the air. The blast effect is rare compared to the high-voltage effect of lightning but when it occurs there may be severe wounds, fractures and ruptured eardrums.

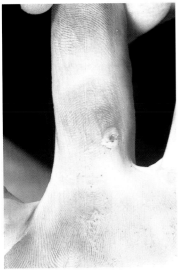

Fig. 39 Subtle example of electrical burn.

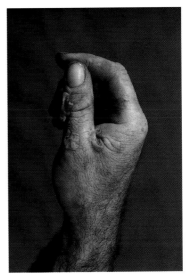

Fig. 40 Electrical burns.

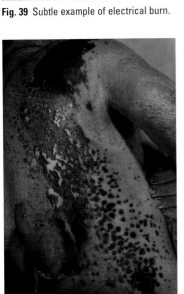

Fig. 41 'Crocodile-skin' appearance in lightning fatality.

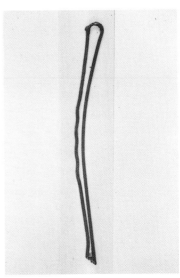

Fig. 42 Hairpin damaged by lightning. The body showed no marks at all.

Stab wounds

Definition The stab wound is a penetrating injury which has, in general, a greater depth in the body than the size of the wound on the body surface.

Features Typically, stab wounds are made with a knife or knives but broken bottles (Fig. 43), implements such as hayforks (Fig. 44), tools such as screwdrivers and household items such as scissors may be used. Infrequently, the skin wound appearance may be highly suggestive of a particular weapon, particularly in cases where the same weapon has been used repeatedly.

In clothed bodies, it should be remembered that folds in material may produce an apparent discrepancy between the number of holes in a garment and the number of wounds seen on the skin. Another source of confusion, especially to a jury, is that a knife with a blade of a certain width produces a skin wound which is described in terms of how long it is.

Not infrequently, the same weapon used to create the stab wound may inflict slash wounds on the body, often on the hands (defence injuries) (Fig. 45).

The physical properties of the skin, the dynamic nature of the stabbing process and the rocking or tangential motion of the knife frequently produce apparent discrepancies between the size of the weapon and the size of the wounds. In general, when several knives are presented as a possible weapon, one can be fairly certain about which did not inflict the injuries.

Description Description of stab wounds should include:

1. Dimensions of surface wounds—the edges of each wound are apposed to record a length.
2. Position and orientation of the stab wounds, including distance from fixed reference points such as the midline and the heels.
3. The structures penetrated by the stab wounds and the dimensions of wounds in these structures. Organs such as the liver or kidney may provide useful evidence of the taper of a penetrating weapon (Fig. 46).
4. The overall direction of thrust.

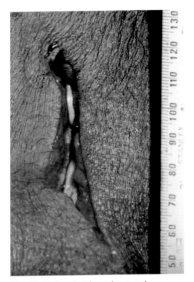

Fig. 43 Broken bottle stab wound.

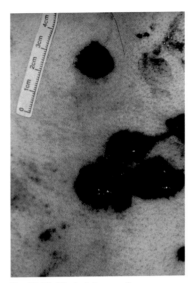

Fig. 44 Pitchfork stab wounds.

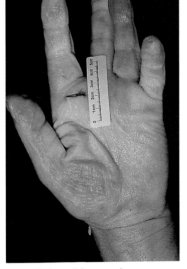

Fig. 45 Defence injury to palm.

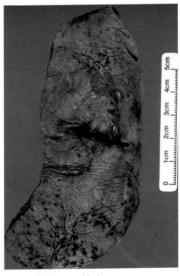

Fig. 46 Stab wound in lung.

It is important to remember that stabbing a person is a dynamic process, often involving two persons who are moving relative to each other. Over-interpretation of the evidence is to be avoided.

Weapon examination

The pathologist may be asked to examine the alleged weapon, be it knife, gun or any other implement that can inflict injury.

The weapon is treated as a potentially infective source for diseases such as hepatitis.

The pathologist should also be careful to avoid contamination of the alleged weapon. The examination of the weapon should be separate from the examination of the injuries.

Cutting weapons

Examination

Important information obtained from the scrutiny of the weapon includes:

1. dimensions (Fig. 47)—length, width and thickness of blade if a knife is submitted
2. sharpness of tip and of edge(s)
3. number of cutting edges and any particular properties of those cutting edges
4. the shape of the hilt guard.

The sharpness of the tip of the weapon is the most important factor in skin penetration (Fig. 48). Once the skin has been breached, penetration to the hilt is obtainable with minimal force, provided there is no skeletal tissue in the way. Bone or calcified cartilage is a greater barrier to a weapon's entry than skin, and penetration of those materials implies a greater force.

Knifemarks in skeletal tissue

The approximate length, blade width and sharpness of a knife may be suggested on examination of skeletal remains. In thoracic stabbings, a cutting edge in a rib (Fig. 49) or costal cartilage is a useful finding. Knife marks on costal cartilage have identifiable features that can be accurately replicated using dental impression material. Figure 50 shows multiple termination marks on the femur from a multiple stabbing case.

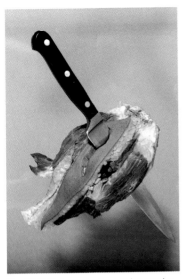

Fig. 47 Knife in excised wound; note size of surface wound.

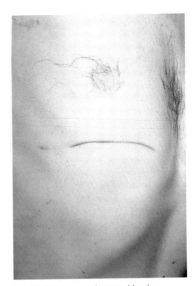

Fig. 48 Slash wound caused by tip.

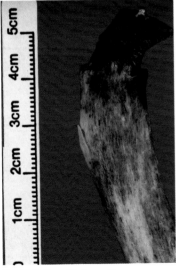

Fig. 49 Knife cut to bony rib.

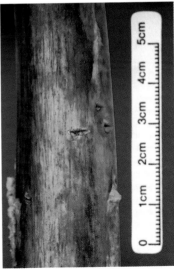

Fig. 50 Stab wounds to femur.

Guns

Examination

Many pathologists prefer to leave the examination of a gun to the ballistics expert. It is, however, useful to know the dimensions and calibre of the gun.

Classification

Guns can be classified simply into those that fire a single projectile and those that fire a collection of small projectiles, for example lead shot. The former include rifles, which may use high- or low-velocity ammunition, and pistols, while shotguns are an example of the latter.

Autopsy findings
(Figs 51–54)

As with any injury, examination of the body may suggest the probable type of weapon that caused the injury. In firearm injuries, the site of the wound and the range of discharge are important in helping to decide whether the death is suicide, accident or homicide. Classical sites of election for firearm suicide are:

- forehead
- temple
- mouth
- precordium.

Contact firearm injuries in these sites do not exclude homicide, however. Scene of crime examination and careful police investigation are essential.

In suicide, it is to be expected that the weapon should be found at the death scene, but its absence does not absolutely exclude suicide.

Examination of clothing

An entrance hole in clothing, if made by a lead or a full metal-jacketed bullet, may demonstrate a grey to black rim known as 'bullet wipe'. The material deposited consists of grease, soot and debris from the barrel of the gun. This same material is wiped onto the skin of an entrance wound, if the person shot is unclothed.

The pathologist may be asked to comment on the distance between the muzzle of the firearm and the body when the firearm was discharged. This question should be treated with caution and a few generalizations made. As with the examination of the gun, the scientific investigation of distance is more properly the domain of the ballistics expert.

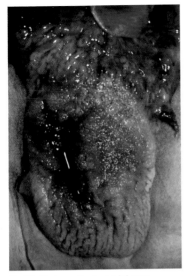

Fig. 51 Shotgun discharge injury to tongue.

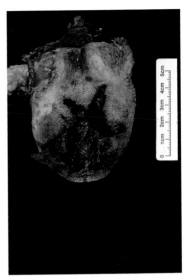

Fig. 52 Handgun discharge injury to tongue in putrefied case.

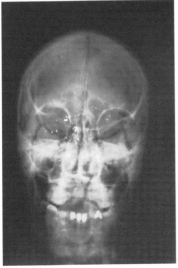

Fig. 53 X-ray of skull in handgun suicide.

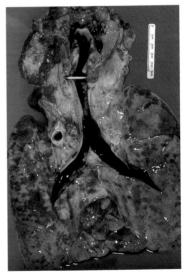

Fig. 54 Aspiration of blood associated with gunshot facial injuries.

Gunshot wounds

Single projectile The appearance of a gunshot wound caused by a single projectile varies according to range. The following general features apply:

Contact wound (0–2 cm)
- Ragged entrance wound if overlying bone.
- Soot/powder deposition obvious macroscopically (Fig. 55).
- Carbon monoxide in tissues.

Close range (2–50 cm)
- Circular wound which is likely to be inverted.
- Soot/powder deposition (tattooing) often only detectable microscopically (Fig. 56).
- Singed hairs/abrasion collar.

Longer range
- Inverted, abraded, circular wound.
- Grease soiling from the bullet.
- Absence of powder/soot macroscopically and microscopically.

A low-velocity projectile may have insufficient energy to exit (Fig. 57), especially if it hits bony structures (Fig. 58).

Shotguns The general features of shotgun wounds are described below. Infrequently, the discharge from a shotgun may strike the body at a tangent, producing a wound that may be mistaken for a laceration.

Contact
- Rounded hole with narrow rim of soot.
- Carbon monoxide in tissues.

Close range
- Round or oval hole with tendency to have a ragged margin.
- Soot deposition/singeing of hair.

Longer range. Increased range allows divergence of the lead shot, producing a central hole with peripheral tiny separated holes. Eventually, the central hole disappears and leaves a scattering of small holes. Measurement of the diameter of the scatter pattern can be used to give an approximate range, subject to ballistic testing with the actual gun.

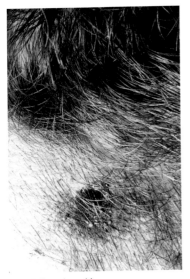

Fig. 55 Soot deposition.

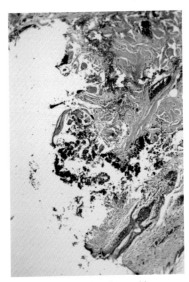

Fig. 56 Soot deposition detectable microscopically.

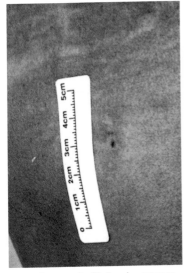

Fig. 57 Spent projectile in subcutaneous position.

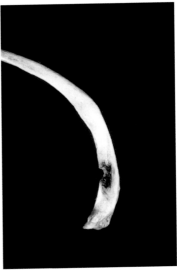

Fig. 58 Projectile injury to rib.

Firearm injuries

Description As with other types of wounds, firearm injuries should be described with reference to fixed anatomical points, particularly the heels and the midline. Trajectory is also important and, in general, is usually a straight line from entry to exit or to projectile. Lateral (Fig. 59) and anterior–posterior X-rays are essential.

Associated features Contact and close range discharge of a shotgun at the head commonly cause extensive destruction of the head, including the entrance wound. The constituents of the shotgun cartridge, such as cardboard and plastic wad, are not infrequently found in the wound (Fig. 60).

Firearms, applied at contact or close range, may also recoil to produce a wound adjacent to the main entrance wound. This recoil injury is typically in the form of an abrasion or bruise.

Blood and tissue from a contact wound may be blasted back into the barrel of the firearm, an event known as 'back spatter'. Back spatter may also cause similar materials to be deposited on the hand of the person firing the weapon.

Estimation of range with shotguns can be made with a better degree of accuracy than for single-projectile weapons.

Figure 61 shows an example of a homicidal shotgun wound to the back. The peripheral separate holes caused by the diversion of lead shot can be seen. Figure 62 shows the lead shot that had accumulated in the chest. The heart was severely lacerated and its chambers shredded by the discharge of lead shot.

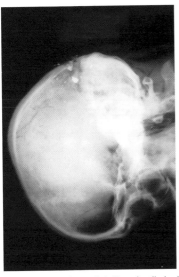

Fig. 59 Lateral X-ray of skull; projectile had exited at the occiput.

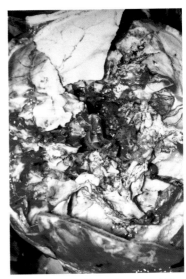

Fig. 60 Plastic wad from shotgun cartridge amidst fragmented base of skull.

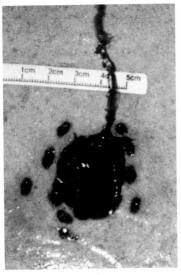

Fig. 61 Shotgun wound.

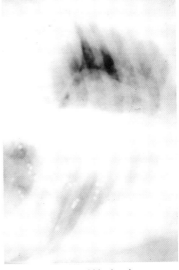

Fig. 62 Lead shot within the chest (X-ray).

Miscellaneous patterned injuries

Stomping   Stomping or kicking injuries are common in a pub brawl and they, not uncommonly, have complications that lead to death. Head trauma may be complicated by intracranial haemorrhage or by aspiration of blood from fractured facial bones (see Fig. 54, p. 32).

Trauma to the head may cause acute injury to mid-line structures of the brain, such as septum pellucidum and periventricular areas. Figure 63 shows acute injuries of this type in a female who received a severe kicking to the head. The septum pellucidum is torn and bloodstained ventricular contents were noted. There are also small, but significant, periventricular haemorrhages.

Jumping on the chest may cause extensive rib fractures, pneumothorax and visceral injury. Jumping on the abdomen causes many similar injuries to the abdominal injuries described for children (see p. 65). Intra-abdominal haemorrhage and also evacuation of faeces are common findings in adult abdominal trauma.

Hand injuries   It may be alleged that the deceased had been involved in a fight prior to his demise. X-ray of the hands may demonstrate one or more fractured metacarpals as evidence that he may have been punching somebody or something.

The skin over the heads of the metacarpals should also be incised, at autopsy, to look for bruising (Fig. 64).

Drag marks   Homicide may be followed by attempts at disposal or hiding of a body. The unclothed body may demonstrate parallel grooved abrasions, typically on the most prominent areas of the back (Fig. 65) as the feet are pulled along. Such marks can be very subtle. Drag marks, of course, may occur on any skin surface in contact with a roughened area.

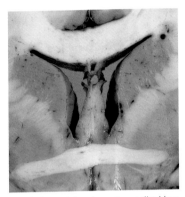

Fig. 63 Acute injury to septum pellucidum and adjacent area of the brain.

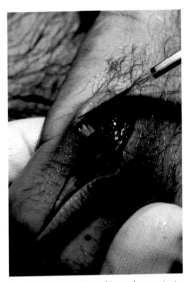

Fig. 64 Incision of knuckle to demonstrate bruising.

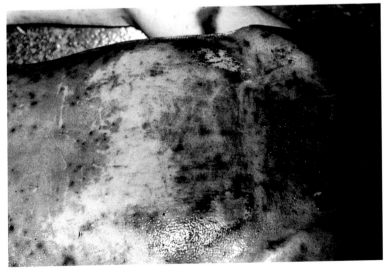

Fig. 65 Drag marks.

9 / **Injuries to bone**

Bone is a hard-wearing substance and may demonstrate the evidence of previous trauma long after the soft tissues have disappeared. Penetration of bone is frequently associated with the application of severe force and this rule particularly applies to stab wounds. The weapon used to produce the stab wounds may indent or cut a bone but fracture is unusual.

Child abuse Accidental fractures of the ribs are uncommon in children and such fractures should be viewed with suspicion, especially if the fractures appear to be of different ages. Injuries around the metaphyses and epiphyses of growing bones, diaphyseal spinal fracture of a long bone and skull fractures may also be seen in child abuse. Medical conditions predisposing to fracture, such as osteogenesis imperfecta (brittle bone disease), syphilis, spina bifida and other conditions should be excluded. It is also important to exclude steroid therapy.

Blunt instrument Applied force with a blunt instrument usually provides a variable pattern of fractures depending on the weight of the weapon, the force used and the number of blows. Comminuted depressed fractures may occur and, in the skeletonized remains, the skull may be fragmented. In blunt head injury there may be accompanying fractures in the bones of the hands (Fig. 66). Such fractures are a variety of defence injury and reflect attempts by the deceased to try to protect the head.

Some weapons may leave a recognizable pattern (Fig. 67). A hammer may produce a circular, partly depressed fracture. Axes inflict wedge-shaped slices if the cutting edge is used, or oblong wounds if the back is used. Radiating linear fractures commonly accompany such injuries.

Animals Some animals leave characteristic bite marks on bone. The saltwater crocodile, for example, which is common in Northern Australia, leaves conical indentations, typically in the extremities. The diameter of the indentations and their distance apart can be employed to estimate the size of the animal (Figs 68 & 69). The digestive juices of the crocodile form an effective decalcifying agent. Crocodiles have occasionally been used as convenient disposal agents for homicide victims.

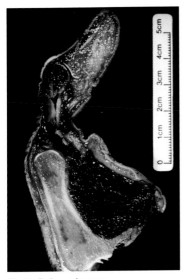

Fig. 66 Defence fracture.

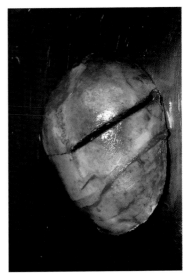

Fig. 67 Dutch hoe injury to skull.

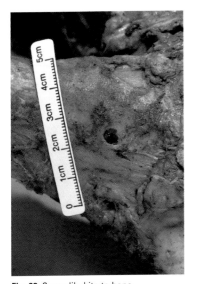

Fig. 68 Crocodile bite to bone.

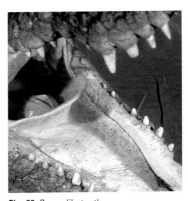

Fig. 69 Crocodile teeth.

Natural disease A wide spectrum of natural diseases may be seen in skeletal remains, particularly osteoarthritis, the most common form of arthritis. Diseased bones are useful in both identification and in trying to establish the age of skeletal remains. In ancient Aboriginal remains, the lesions of yaws are not uncommon (Fig. 70).

Shotgun injury Extensive fractures are usual.

Indentations consistent with the size of the shot in the cartridge may be found in bone (Fig. 71). Occasionally, shot is embedded in the bone.

Cratering The passage of a projectile through the skull produces a phenomenon known as 'cratering' or 'bevelling'. This phenomenon describes the shape of the entrance (Fig. 72) and exit (Fig. 73) wounds in the skull. The projectile drills through the outer table of the skull and removes a cone-shaped bony area from between the outer and inner tables of the skull. The process of cratering continues as the projectile hits the other side of the skull so that another cone-shaped area of bone is removed (see diagram below).

The areas of cratering are commonly different for exit and entrance wounds.

Cratering of the skull

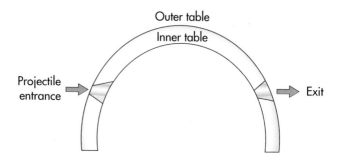

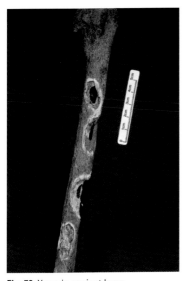

Fig. 70 Yaws in ancient bone.

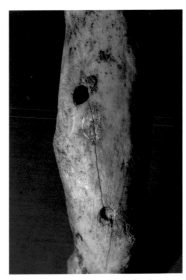

Fig. 71 Lead shot indentations in rib.

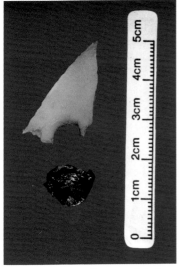

Fig. 72 Soot on entry fragment of skull.
Retrieved deformed bullet also shown.

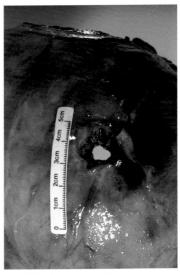

Fig. 73 Cratering in an exit wound.

Post-mortem predation

Animal attack on a corpse is not uncommon, especially in subtropical and tropical climates. The main culprits are insects, crabs, fish and certain predatory mammals. The insect activity may sometimes be useful in assessing when the death occurred.

Features In general, post-mortem predation is usually easy to recognize because of:

- a lack of tissue reaction to the animal injuries
- a tendency to involve areas not covered by clothing.

The main problem caused by post-mortem predation is that wounds inflicted in life may attract attention for the animal attack and artefacts may thus be created. In head injury, for example, animal attack may cause scattering of skull fragments around a sizeable area. Pets are an occasional source of post-mortem mutilation.

In most parts of the world, it is to be expected that local wild animals are capable of post-mortem predation. In the Queensland bush in Australia, for example, the main mammals causing post-mortem predation are feral pigs (Fig. 74), foxes and dingoes. Reptiles such as crocodiles and goannas may also feed on human remains.

Animal attack causing death

There are large numbers of animals that may attack and kill man. Many of these animals are found in Australia and certain examples are discussed below.

Jellyfish stings Marine jellyfish may cause a variety of unpleasant effects, including death. Envenomation is not uncommon in Southern waters where the Pacific box jellyfish (*Chironex fleckeri*) is indigenous. *Chiropsalmus* and *Carybdea* species may also cause deaths, especially in children. In the Northern Hemisphere, cases of sudden fatal reaction have been caused most frequently by the Portuguese man-of-war (*Physalia physalis*).

The box jellyfish has been described as the 'world's most venomous animal'. The toxin is injected by nematocysts into the skin and has both dermatonecrotic and cardiotoxic properties. 4 metres of tentacle contact can cause death.

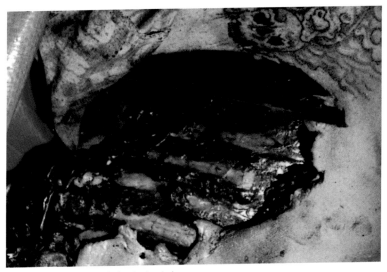

Fig. 74 Post-mortem predation by feral pig.

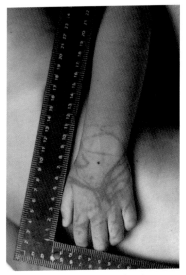

Fig. 75 Box jellyfish injury to hand.

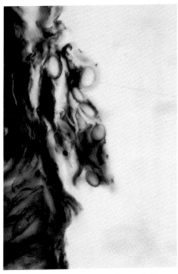

Fig. 76 Nematocysts on surface of skin.

Fatal cases demonstrate multiple linear tentacle marks which look like whip wheals. The hands are typically involved (Fig. 75). Histology of the skin reveals thread portions of the discharged nematocyst tubes penetrating epidermis and papillary dermis (Fig. 76).

Snake bite

The fangs usually inflict two puncture holes, several millimetres apart, at each strike. The venom may be neurotoxic or it may injure muscle (Fig. 77). The other effects of snake venom include a coagulopathy. Cerebral haemorrhage may be found at autopsy and it is sometimes noted that post-mortem clots are absent.

Snake venom contains relatively stable proteins which may be detectable in tissue, provided bacterial infection or putrefaction are absent. Venom detection kits are available commercially. Urinary venom may remain detectable even though the snake bite victim has received antivenom treatment. The bitten area of skin is the best source of material for venom detection. Regional lymph nodes may also be used.

Bee/wasp stings

Bee and wasp stings on the skin may be extremely difficult to identify at autopsy (Fig. 78). Histological sections of the larynx may demonstrate oedema associated with anaphylaxis. Blood samples should be taken for measurement of serum tryptase, IgE and for other evidence of atopy.

Serum tryptase levels are an indicator of mast cell activation and suggest, if elevated, an allergic mediator release, particularly in anaphylaxis. Blood samples should be taken as soon as possible after the death, preferably within 4 hours.

Mosquito bites

Worldwide, mosquitoes are important vectors of malaria (Fig. 79), which can present with many and varying symptoms. Cerebral malaria is a frequent cause of death in untreated cases. Mosquitoes spread yellow fever in certain parts of Africa and tropical America. Mosquito bites are notorious in Australia for their role in outbreaks of dengue, epidemic polyarthritis (Ross River fever) and other arbovirus infections. Fatalities are infrequently seen by forensic pathologists.

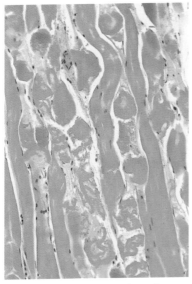

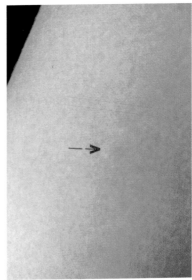

Fig. 77 Coagulative necrosis of muscle at site of snake bite.

Fig. 78 Wasp sting.

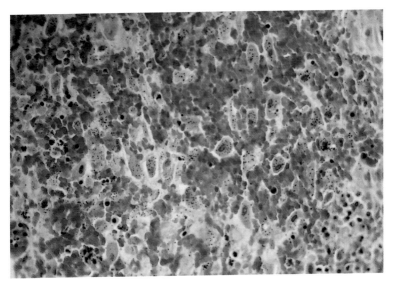

Fig. 79 Malarial pigment in decidual cells.

Crocodile attacks

Australian crocodiles cause injuries that are not dissimilar to those inflicted by alligators or crocodiles in other parts of the world.

Injuries inflicted by saltwater crocodiles are of two distinct types. The bite may involve a limb and typically it causes crushing and twisting injury to that limb (Fig. 80). The claws of the crocodile, by contrast, inflict linear lacerations that may be confused with incised wounds (Fig. 81).

Figure 82 shows a set of bones involved in a crocodile attack. The white-coloured bones were recovered from the stomach of a crocodile and form a partly digested ankle and foot. They are compared to skeletal fragments of leg that were previously found on the bank of the creek.

Spider bites

The majority of spiders produce venom but only certain spiders can bite humans. It is important to remember that death may occur as a result of introduced infection rather than as a consequence of introduced venom. It cannot be overstated that there is a common danger from infection resulting from any break in the skin whether it be from spider bite, bee sting, sharp plant or jagged metal. It has been demonstrated that a variety of common organisms such as several species of *Bacillus*, coagulase-negative *Staphylococcus* and *Penicillium* are contained in spider venom.

Individuals with allergies may react severely to spider venom. Spider fangs leave two puncture marks on the victim's skin (Fig. 83). The adjacent skin is typically erythematous and oedematous. At autopsy, such a bite can be removed with a margin of undamaged skin for venom studies or culture.

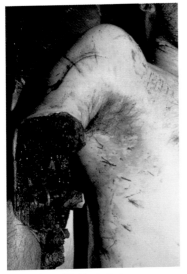

Fig. 80 Crocodile bite to limb.

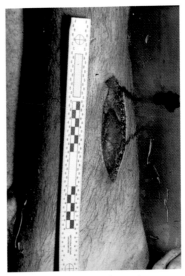

Fig. 81 Crocodile claw injury to leg.

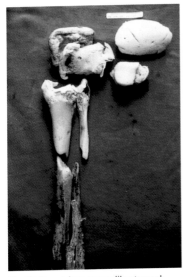

Fig. 82 Bones from crocodile stomach and leg bones from bank of creek.

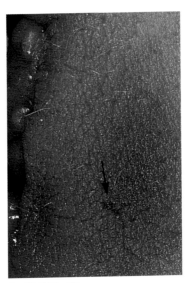

Fig. 83 Spider bite.

Shark bites   Shark bites may be encountered in victims who have been swimming in fresh water far upstream from the sea, as well as in estuarine and marine situations. The details of the bite vary with the causative species.

During the process of biting, the bottom jaw tends to hook into and fix the location of the prey, while the victim is shaken against the top jaw which scythes from side to side. This results in a clean-cut bite with a characteristic appearance. The size of the bite, the 'bite radius', can be linked to the size of the animal causing the wound (Fig. 84).

The most common cause of death is from hypovolaemic shock following the attack. Analysis of fatal cases occurring in Queensland has shown that bite marks to the thigh area are seen most frequently (Fig. 85). Certain victims display just one fatal injury while others may demonstrate multiple areas of damage, with missing limbs (Fig. 86).

Fragments of tooth embedded in the wounds can frequently lead to identification of the species responsible. In Australian waters, the whaler sharks, the tiger shark (*Galeocerdo cuvier*) and the great white shark (*Carcharodon carcharias*) are common offenders.

Sharks may also feed on bodies after death (post-mortem predation) and it may be impossible to determine whether the injuries are the cause of death or not (Fig. 87). In the case illustrated, the prosthetic device on the leg was a valuable aid to identification.

Ticks   Ticks, when left to their own devices, do not normally cause death in humans. The act of squeezing a tick during attempted removal may result in tick fluids passing into the host and triggering a fatal anaphylactic shock.

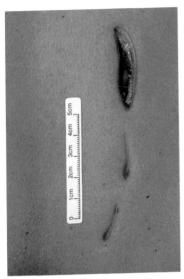

Fig. 84 Shark bite mark.

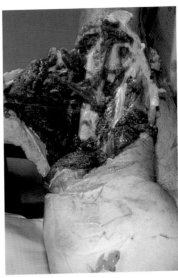

Fig. 85 Shark bite to thigh.

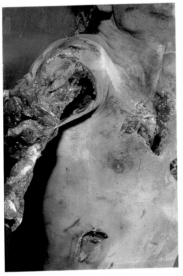

Fig. 86 Limb removal by shark.

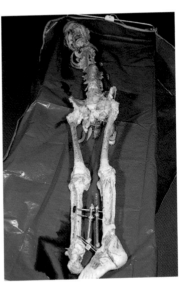

Fig. 87 Probable post-mortem shark attack.

11 / **Natural disease**

Sudden deaths attributable to natural disease comprise the bulk of the cases seen by forensic pathologists. Certain of such deaths will be considered under three main systems: cardiovascular, respiratory and central nervous system. In any suspicious or unnatural death, the significance of, and any contribution from, natural disease, requires to be assessed.

Cardiovascular system

Definitions

Aneurysm. An aneurysm is a localized area of ballooning in the wall of a vessel. Ruptured atheromatous aneurysms are a common cause of death in those parts of the world where ischaemic heart disease occurs. Atheromatous aneurysms usually occur below the diaphragm but infrequently they can be in the thorax, in which site they should be distinguished from syphilitic aneurysms.

Myocardial ischaemia. Myocardial ischaemia is one of the commonest causes of death worldwide and is a direct result of impaired supply of oxygenated blood to the myocardium.

Myocardial infarction. Myocardial infarction is the death (necrosis) of myocardium caused by an inadequate supply of oxygenated blood to the myocardium. It is a consequence of sustained myocardial ischaemia (Figs 88, 89 & 90).

Causes of myocardial ischaemia or infarction. Most myocardial infarcts occur in hearts supplied by arteries demonstrating severe complicated atheroma (Fig. 91). Angiographic studies have indicated that thrombus developing on ulcerated atheromatous plaque is important in producing an acute diminution of blood supply in a coronary artery. Eccentric atheromatous plaque with abundant lipid are prone to rupture and, apart from overlying thrombus, they may demonstrate haemorrhage into the plaque. In most coronial deaths due to coronary artery atheroma (this term being synonymous with coronary atherosclerosis), recent myocardial infarction is not found and death is presumed to be due to an arrhythmia consequent upon myocardial ischaemia.

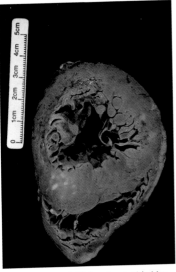

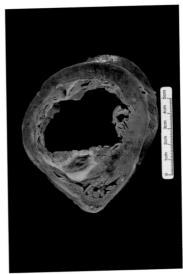

Fig. 88 Myocardial infarction and (white areas) old ischaemic fibrosis.

Fig. 89 Myocardial infarction, mural thrombus and left ventricular failure.

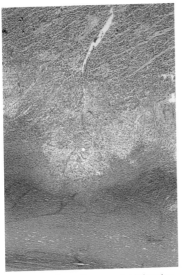

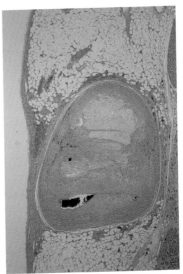

Fig. 90 Histology of myocardial infarction.

Fig. 91 Severe atheroma in coronary artery.

Sudden cardiac death

In sudden cardiac death, examination of the coronary arteries may reveal severe stenosis or thrombosis in a coronary artery (Fig. 91, p. 52). Infrequently, coronary artery dissection is found. Other causes of sudden cardiac death include:

- hypertensive heart disease
- valvular disorders
- cardiomyopathy
- myocarditis
- anomalous or hypoplastic coronary arteries
- coronary artery arteritis
- coronary artery spasm
- coronary artery embolism
- infiltrative diseases
- conduction system defects
- atrial myxoma (Fig. 92).

Valvular heart disease

Floppy mitral valve. In this common condition, accumulation of mucopolysaccharide within the mitral valve cusps produces a ballooned or parachute-like appearance.

When severe, floppy mitral valve may cause mitral incompetence and left ventricular failure. Sudden death may be attributed to floppy mitral valve.

In certain parts of the world, rheumatic fever is an important cause of valvular disease. Figure 93 shows the typical fused chordae of rheumatic valvular disease.

Endocarditis. Microorganisms in the bloodstream may infect a heart valve to form vegetations. These friable vegetations may then break off and embolize to various sites, commonly brain, spleen or kidney. Endocarditis is an important complication of drug abuse (see p. 131).

Pericardial abnormalities

Soldier's plaques. White plaques on the epicardial surface of the heart (Fig. 94) are commonly seen at autopsy and they can be considered to have no relevance to the death.

Carcinomatous pericarditis. Figure 95 shows a subtle example of carcinomatous pericarditis. In such cases, the pericardial fluid is usually haemorrhagic.

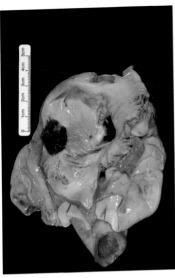

Fig. 92 Atrial myxoma.

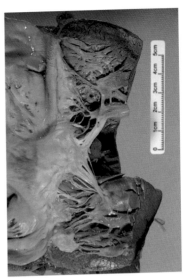

Fig. 93 Fused chordae in rheumatic valvular disease.

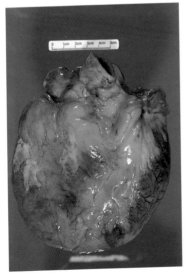

Fig. 94 Epicardial plaques.

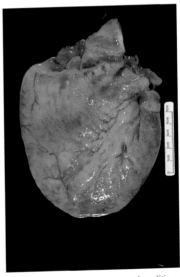

Fig. 95 Early carcinomatous pericarditis.

Respiratory system

Asthma. In recent years, concern has been expressed about the high mortality due to asthma, particularly since many deaths might be avoided. Asthma is a disease characterized by an abrupt onset of narrowing of the bronchial airways. This narrowing can be caused by irritant substances being inhaled, by exposure to an allergen or by emotional stress. Figures 96 and 97 show the use of special stains to show certain histological features of asthma.

There has been a recent interest in the relationship between thunderstorms and asthma. The experience in Brisbane, Australia, where there are frequent thunderstorms, is that they are probably not relevant to asthma fatalities. Asthma deaths are not uncommonly associated with drug abuse, especially when materials are smoked.

Pulmonary thrombo-embolism. This term describes occlusive blood clot in the pulmonary arteries (Fig. 98), the blood clot usually embolic in origin. A deep venous thrombosis (Fig. 99) of the lower limbs is a common source of such emboli. Deep venous thrombosis seldom occurs without some predisposing event or underlying condition, such as myocardial infarction or immobility.

Infection. Infections range from an acute epiglottitis to a florid bronchopneumonia but may all kill quickly. An important public health exercise of the autopsy is to establish the identity of the causative organisms, although this may be difficult in the case of fragile organisms such as the meningococcus and also in the presence of decomposition.

Pneumothorax

This term describes the accumulation of gas, usually air, in the thoracic cavity. It is a complication of many respiratory diseases and also of chest trauma. The condition is easily missed at autopsy and is demonstrable by puncturing the thorax under a pocket of water and checking for the escape of bubbles.

In transportation accidents, there may be treatment of pneumothorax by the insertion of chest drains at hospital. In fatal cases, it is important not to confuse the drain wounds with stab wounds.

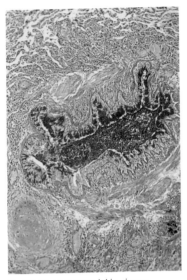

Fig. 96 Mucous material in airway (asthma).

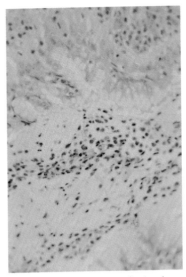

Fig. 97 Eosinophils in airway (asthma).

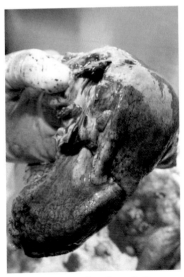

Fig. 98 Pulmonary thrombo-embolism.

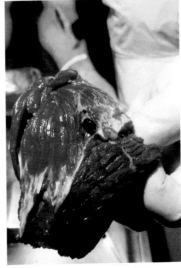

Fig. 99 Deep venous thrombosis.

Central nervous system

Subarachnoid haemorrhage. Non-traumatic subarachnoid haemorrhage is typically produced by rupture of an aneurysm (Fig. 100), usually of berry type or, in older patients, of atheromatous origin. It is advisable to remove the blood from the fresh brain to aid identification of the aneurysm. Failure to find an aneurysm should prompt a search for evidence of a traumatic cause for the subarachnoid haemorrhage. This search should include examination of the neck in the region of the mastoid process and angiography or dissection of the vertebral arteries.

Epilepsy. Epilepsy is characterized by a low threshold for seizures. Hypoxic changes associated with seizures over a long period of time may be detected histologically in the hippocampi of the brain.

Post-mortem examination may yield evidence of a bitten tongue (Fig. 101) and neuropathological abnormalities, but, not infrequently, the diagnosis may have to be made by exclusion of other causes of death. Histological examination of the tongue can effectively demonstrate recent bruising caused by biting and may also reveal evidence of previous such trauma. The tongue is sometimes clamped between the teeth in rigor mortis and this appearance should *not* be interpreted as evidence of epilepsy.

Cerebral haemorrhage. Such haemorrhages are usually immediately obvious in the fresh brain at autopsy, especially when the haemorrhage is in an important area such as the pons (Fig. 102). Problems may arise in motor vehicle accidents when the haemorrhage may have preceded a fatal crash with severe head injury. Fixation of the brain and dissection by a neuropathologist may resolve some of these problems.

Colloid cyst of the third ventricle. This is a rare cause of sudden death which may be heralded by headaches. The cyst is an example of how a simple, non-malignant structure can kill because of its location in a crucial site (Fig. 103). The cyst may be missed if the brain is sectioned in the fresh state.

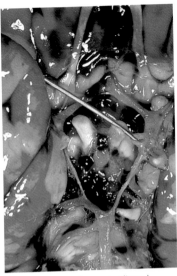

Fig. 100 Rupture of saccular (berry) aneurysm.

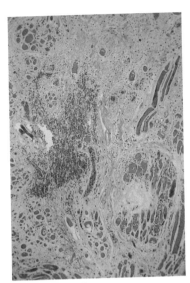

Fig. 101 Bruising in tongue.

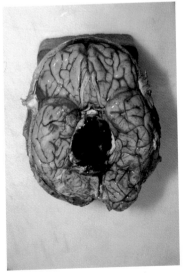

Fig. 102 Primary pontine haemorrhage.

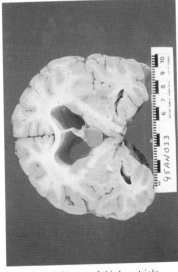

Fig. 103 Colloid cyst of third ventricle.

12 / **Deaths in infants**

An infant is a child of under 1 year. One of the more common causes of death in this group is sudden infant death syndrome (SIDS).

SIDS

This cause of death is diagnosed by exclusion of all other possible causes of death. The aetiology of SIDS is not known but, currently, abnormalities of wakefulness/respiration receptors in the brain stem are suspected.

Clinical features
- Peak incidence between 2 and 4 months of age.
- Increased risk in twins.
- Increased risk in cold season; April to September in Australia (Fig. 104).
- More common in temperate and cold areas.
- Smoking in the parental home is a risk factor.
- Breast-feeding may protect babies.
- Infant sleeping in the prone (face down) position is at increased risk.

Cot death

The term cot death includes cases of SIDS and also sudden unexpected deaths which can be explained.

Investigations
History. There may be information on how sudden the death actually was and also on any congenital abnormalities or acquired disease demonstrated by the infant. Was there resuscitation and for how long?

Scene. It is not uncommon, in our experience, to see blood-tinged fluid in the cot and on the face of the SIDS victim.

Post-mortem examination. A meticulous autopsy is required, starting with a thorough external examination looking for evidence of the stigmata of congenital abnormalities such as abnormal palmar creases (Fig. 105) or malrotated, low-set ears. In the newborn, there may be evidence of distress manifest as meconium staining of the skin and this may be associated with meconium aspiration (Fig. 106).

The body is also scrutinized for external signs of disease or trauma.

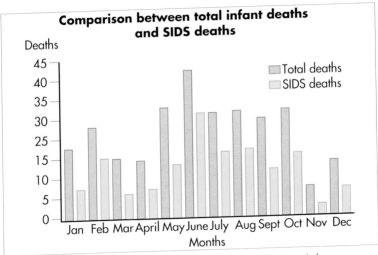

Fig. 104 Monthly infant deaths in Queensland, Australia, over a 5-year period.

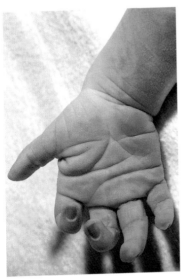

Fig. 105 Abnormal palmar creases.

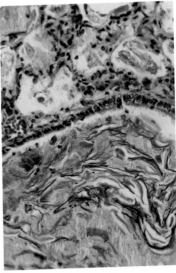

Fig. 106 Meconium aspiration.

Resuscitation artefacts

Pathologists should be aware of the complications of resuscitation. In infants, a variety of significant injuries linked to the application of cardiopulmonary resuscitation have been described. In our experience, chest wall fractures are virtually never seen in infants as their chest wall is supple; we would be very hesitant to attribute such injuries to resuscitation. There are descriptions in the literature, however, of injuries which include not only broken bones and traumatized organs but sometimes superficial soft tissue damage resulting from ventilatory procedures. Such soft tissue injury may make it difficult to distinguish subtle clues suggestive of smothering.

Shaken baby syndrome

It is important to look for evidence of the shaken baby syndrome. This evidence consists of a triad of signs: subdural haematoma, retinal haemorrhages and haemorrhages in the spinal cord (see p. 111).

Radiology

X-ray examination of an infant is one of the most important investigations and may be employed to detect abuse (see p. 39), congenital abnormalities and acquired disease. An abnormal shape to the heart may suggest congenital heart disease.

Cardiovascular system

It is important to be aware of the normal morphology of the cardiac structures before examination of the heart. It is also good practice to dissect the heart while it remains in continuity with the lungs (Fig. 107).

Findings

There may be internal evidence of active disease, mishap (Fig. 108), congenital abnormality (Fig. 109) or trauma (Fig. 110). There should be extensive sampling of tissue for histology.

Other investigations

Biochemistry. Investigation such as vitreous humour glucose estimation may be of value.

Toxicology. Hypnotics and/or alcohol may occasionally be used as infant sedatives.

Microbiology. Investigations should include blood and cerebrospinal fluid culture, viral tissue culture and serology.

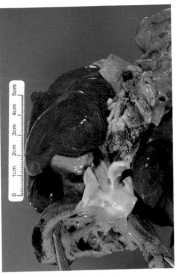

Fig. 107 Univentricular heart.

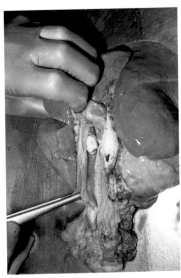

Fig. 108 Foreign body in airway.

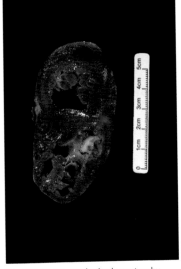

Fig. 109 Right ventricular hypertrophy.

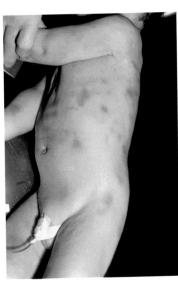

Fig. 110 Infant abuse.

13 / Deaths in children

Consideration of the circumstances of death and of any clinical history is very important in the investigation of childhood deaths, as with any autopsy. Bruises are invariably found in any mobile child and it is important to distinguish between what is within the 'normal' spectrum of childhood bruising and what is abnormal. Medical conditions occasionally mimic bruising and true bruising may be excessive in certain haematological disorders.

Child abuse

Clinical features   In non-accidental injury to a child certain features should be looked for:

- Bruising in unusual places.
- Multiple injuries, especially if of different ages.
- Derangement of the teeth and frenulum damage.
- Bite marks.
- Unusual injuries such as cigarette burns (Fig. 111), scalds (Fig. 158, p. 98), straight-line areas of damage.
- Skeletal damage, especially if of different ages. It is important to be aware of any bone disease in the child and to look for evidence of natural bone disease.

Skin bruising is the most common injury in child abuse (Fig. 112). Frequently, individual bruises may have a size consistent with the forceful application of a prodding finger and clusters of such bruises may be seen in gripping injuries.

The child may have been gripped at a convenient 'handle', for example at the elbow or at the ankle. Incision of the skin not infrequently demonstrates bruising that is not apparent on the surface of the skin. However, gripping injuries are not always seen.

Similarly, reflection of the scalp of the child at post-mortem examination may reveal bruises that were not visible externally on the head (Fig. 113). In young children and infants, diastasis is sometimes seen as a consequence of head injury. Diastasis refers to the separation of skull plates, with or without fractures.

All injuries should be photographed, ideally in colour.

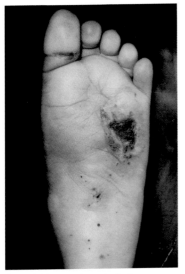

Fig. 111 Cigarette burns to foot.

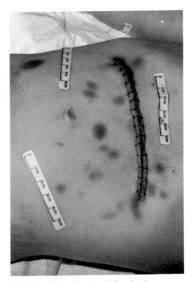

Fig. 112 Abdominal prodding bruises.

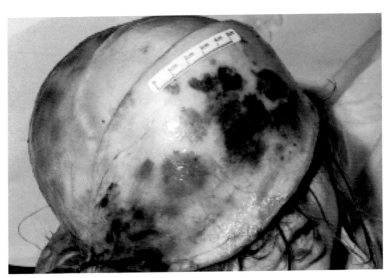

Fig. 113 Reflection of scalp to show recent bruises.

Causes of death   **Head injury.** Slaps to the side of the head may cause bruising of the ears. Occasionally, grip marks may be seen on the face; they form an important record of the size of the hand maintaining the grip.

The skull may demonstrate fracture, depending on the amount of force applied. Children occasionally demonstrate severe fracturing of the skull caused by being thrown against walls or by being battered with a blunt instrument, such as a piece of wood (Fig. 114). In such cases, the brain may show severe disruption similar in extent to motor vehicle accidents. Radiological investigation of the head injury has a number of benefits:

- A permanent record of the injuries is made.
- It provides information on the pathology of injury.
- It alerts the pathologist to the possible existence of abnormal bone.
- It may demonstrate previous bone injury.
- The X-ray can be shown to a jury without causing the distaste that a photograph of the head injuries would cause.

Abdominal injury. This complication is the second commonest cause of death in child abuse after head injury. Injuries seen may include:

- haemoperitoneum following vascular damage; histology may reveal evidence of previous trauma to the vascular pedicles
- laceration in solid organs such as liver or spleen
- peritonitis following intestinal injury.

It is important to document any injuries that are relevant to the death (Fig. 115) and to document any artefacts that may be linked to resuscitation.

Abdominal injuries are occasionally attributed, by defence counsel, to too vigorous resuscitation. Such injuries are rarely due to this cause in our experience.

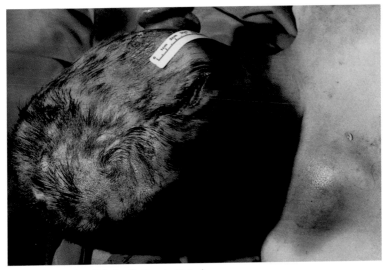

Fig. 114 Severe head injuries (battered with log).

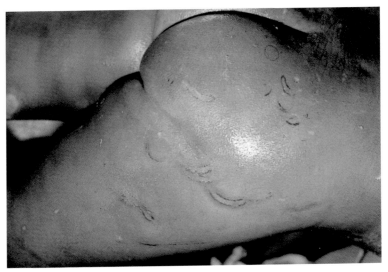

Fig. 115 Belt buckle injuries.

Dog bites

Human bites are relatively common in child abuse and the perpetrator may blame the family dog. A swab of the wound may indicate human saliva rather than canine. The shape of the wound is also likely to be very different for canine teeth, especially in large dogs, although smaller dogs with a more circular bite can produce a wound that is more difficult to differentiate.

Infrequently, fatalities are caused by the attack of a dog or pack of dogs.

Site   Death is particularly liable to occur when the blood vessels of the neck are penetrated or torn. The blood volume in a child is small compared to that of an adult and a dangerous degree of exsanguination can occur quickly.

The face (Fig. 116) is also a potential target for the dog bite and, when large strips of scalp are torn away, there may be problems in identification. Bites are often found on the limbs, particularly the hands, which are attempting to hold the dog away (defence injuries). Figure 117 shows an example of a dingo bite to the thigh. Dingoes and other wild animals may approach humans not uncommonly, especially if encouraged to do so by being thrown scraps.

Dog bites are found in parts of the body that are available for the dog to bite. This depends on the position of the victim; a small child is easily pulled to the ground by a large dog.

Distinguishing features   The dog bite is distinguished by the presence of obvious canine (eye) teeth. These teeth leave wounds that are punctured in appearance, and may sometimes look like abrasions. The other anterior teeth may often not reach the tissues, and so may not leave visible wounds.

Measurement of the inter-canine distance can indicate the size of the dog that inflicted the wound. The size of the dog is also reflected by the size of the holes in the wounds.

Bite marks should usually be photographed both in black and white, and in colour.

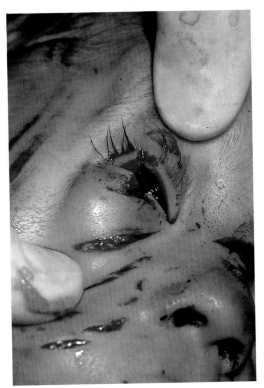

Fig. 116 Dog bite to the face of a child.

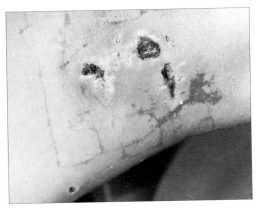

Fig. 117 Dingo bite to the thigh of a child. (Photograph courtesy of Queensland Newspapers.)

Sudden death in children

Certain of the commoner conditions causing sudden death in children will be considered for cardiovascular and respiratory systems.

Cardiovascular system

Infection is very common in childhood and septicaemia may result in myocarditis, endocarditis or rheumatic fever. Myocarditis is also a common complication of viral illness, particularly influenza and Coxsackie A. Children with congenital heart disease are at increased risk of fatal infective complications. Occasionally, children die after surgery for congenital heart disease and the complexity of the surgically corrected abnormal heart may require assistance from the surgeon, a paediatric pathologist or a cardiac pathologist.

Cardiomyopathy and valvular disorders occur in childhood but, in our experience, present rarely as coronial cases.

Respiratory system

Children with neurological problems are particularly prone to aspiration of food into the lungs. They, and also children without neurological problems, are also potentially at risk of obstruction of the upper airways by foreign body. An intrinsic condition, such as an inflamed epiglottis, may also produce airway obstruction. There are various rare neurological conditions where chronic constipation is a feature; such children may develop a fatal exogenous lipid pneumonia (Fig. 118) due to inhalation of liquid paraffin.

Other respiratory causes of childhood sudden death include asthma, bronchopneumonia, cystic fibrosis and tension pneumothorax. It may be difficult to appreciate the distension of the lungs in asthma (Fig. 119) if the pathologist does infrequent autopsies on children.

The histological features of asthma can sometimes be very subtle. There may be plugging of bronchi by mucinous material. One of the important features is eosinophils in the mucosal lamina propria with transmigration through the mucosal epithelium into the mucus plug. There is often hypertrophy of smooth muscle around the small airways, usually associated with repeated spasm of these airways. (Certain microscopic features of asthma are shown in Figs 96 & 97, p. 56.)

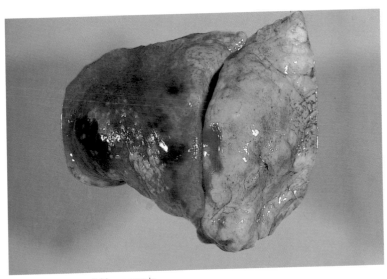

Fig. 118 Exogenous lipid pneumonia.

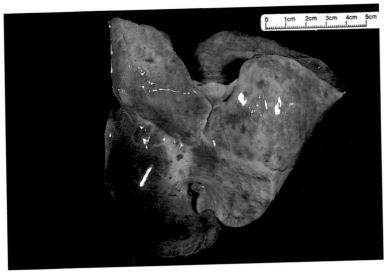

Fig. 119 Asthma.

14 / **Transportation injuries**

Forensic pathologists see transportation deaths frequently, usually in small numbers but occasionally in large numbers (mass disaster). It is important to establish the role of drink, drugs or disease in the cause of accident, especially if the person is in control of the transport. A 'hit and run' death may require the collection of relevant evidence, such as fragments of vehicle or paint and reference blood for grouping and hair, at autopsy.

Pedestrians   Pedestrians, if hit by a car, may demonstrate injuries corresponding to the height of the point of impact. Bumper contact, for example, may produce fractured lower limbs. At autopsy, the distance of such injuries above the heels should be measured for possible comparison with bumper height.

Cyclists   Head injuries are common in cyclists either hit by cars or propelled from their bicycles. Many of the victims are children and there may be diffuse cerebral oedema, often without evidence of skull fracture or scalp injury. Others demonstrate diffuse axonal injury of the brain, with haemorrhages in the corpus callosum and in dorsolateral areas of the rostral brain stem (see p. 115).

Motor cyclists   Motor cyclists may have extensive 'brush abrasions' due to sliding across a road (Fig. 120). They also may demonstrate a 'hinge' fracture, a transverse crack across the middle cranial fossa. Ejection from the bike into signs or fences may cause injuries mimicking seat belt marks (Fig. 121).

Motor vehicle occupants   The driver may demonstrate injuries caused by the steering wheel. The occupants, particularly those in the front seats, may demonstrate facial injuries due to contact with windscreen glass, known as 'sparrow's foot' marks. They also may demonstrate seat belt injuries (Fig. 122) and lacerations or abrasions due to contact with protuberant surfaces. Unrestrained passengers may also demonstrate spinal injuries.

Train over-run   There may be extremely severe disruption of the body in train over-run, often making identification difficult. In Queensland, Australia, approximately half the cases are accidents and are associated with a high blood alcohol level or evidence of drug abuse.

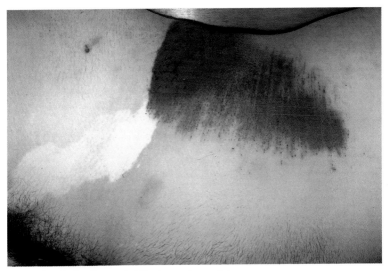

Fig. 120 Brush abrasions and vitiligo in a motor cyclist.

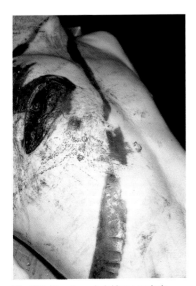

Fig. 121 Abrasion mimicking seat belt injury in a motor cyclist.

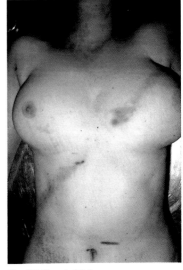

Fig. 122 Seat belt injury.

15 / **Asphyxia**

Definition Asphyxia means absence of pulsation but commonly the term is used to describe deprivation of oxygen (hypoxia) or lack of oxygen (anoxia).

Obstruction to the flow of oxygen occurs at several levels.

Levels **External to the body.** Suffocation will occur if there is insufficient oxygen in the inhaled atmosphere. Smothering is the form of asphyxia which occurs if the nose and mouth are obstructed.

Within the upper airways. The size of the offending object will correspond with the level of obstruction. Materials such as food (Fig. 123), infective debris, tumours, damaged or false teeth and, infrequently, fellated objects may obstruct.

Rigidity of the chest. Traumatic (crush) asphyxia occurs when there is restriction of the respiratory movement of the thorax.

Pulmonary disease. Certain diseases, notably the pneumoconioses and others, such as idiopathic fibrosing alveolitis, may insidiously prevent free gaseous exchange within the lungs.

Circulatory problems. Heart problems may produce severe cardiopulmonary impairment. Anaemia may contribute to such circulatory problems.

Cellular damage. Certain poisons impair the ability of the tissues to use delivered oxygen.

Laryngeal injuries Prolonged intubation produces a typical pattern of laryngeal damage, consisting of mucosal ulceration along the posterior-medial aspects of both vocal cords.

Infective laryngitis. It can be very difficult macroscopically to identify laryngitis and inflammation in adjacent structures in cases of cot death. Widespread histological sampling of this area is recommended as, uncommonly, laryngitis may be the primary focus for a fatal septicaemia.

A diagnosis of infective laryngitis should be supported by microbiological tests. Aspiration of certain poisons, particularly those of corrosive type, may mimic bacterial infection of the airways (Fig. 124).

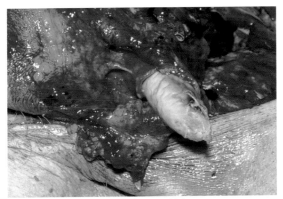

Fig. 123 Sausage impaction in laryngeal inlet.

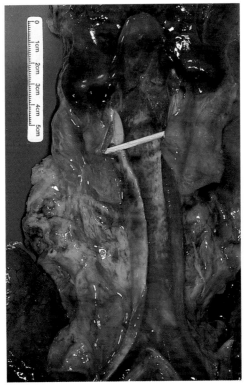

Fig. 124 Inhalation of a corrosive insecticide.

Hanging

Features Hanging causes death by compression of the neck; the compression usually maintained by ligature but occasionally by unusual means such as the forked branch of a tree. The ligature is commonly a rope or a length of wire.

Internal damage to neck structures is usually slight compared to the depth of the hanging mark (Fig. 125). A compressed carotid artery may show intimal tearing (Fig. 126), especially if the artery has complicated atheroma. Infrequently, there are fractures of the hyoid bone and thyroid cartilage. Large amounts of haemorrhage should be viewed with suspicion, especially if there are bruises and unexplained wounds on the neck. Scene examination can be very important in detecting homicide dressed up as suicidal hanging.

Figure 127 shows a female who was suspended by a leather belt after being bashed and strangled. In general, the features to look for include evidence of dragging to the place of suspension, irregularities in the suspension process and also signs of drugging.

In suicidal hanging, complete suspension is not necessary and the feet may be on the ground.

In contrast to strangulation, in hanging the slope of the ligature mark is usually upwards towards the back of the neck. When looking at the back of the neck, an inverted V-shaped mark is often seen, the apex of the V pointing in the general direction of suspension.

Petechiae Petechiae are tiny punctate haemorrhages, typically found in lax tissues such as the eyelid (Fig. 128), but also found elsewhere on the face and neck. They may be seen on larynx, mucous membranes, scalp and on viscera.

Petechiae of the visceral pleura of the lung are classically known as 'Tardieu's spots'. Petechiae are often absent or infrequent in hanging but may be seen in other asphyxial deaths such as traumatic asphyxia, strangulation and throttling.

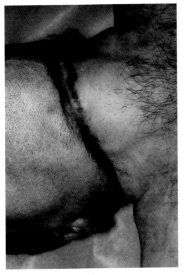

Fig. 125 Hanging mark.

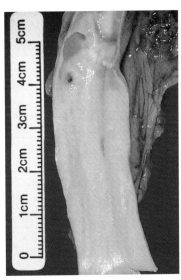

Fig. 126 Intimal tear in carotid artery.

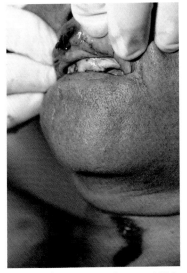

Fig. 127 Homicide dressed up as suicidal hanging.

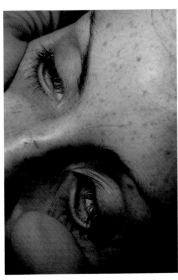

Fig. 128 Petechial haemorrhages in lower eyelids.

Strangulation

Ligature strangulation

The ligature mark is usually a horizontal groove around the neck, typically just above or below the thyroid cartilage. Fractures to the laryngeal cartilages are relatively uncommon. Petechiae, conjunctival haemorrhages and facial cyanosis are common but such signs may be absent if the death has been rapid, as by cardiac inhibition.

A 'Spanish windlass' arrangement is occasionally used for suicidal strangulations such as in Figure 129, the ligature in this case being tightened by winding the hammer.

Strangulation by ligature is mainly homicide and the victim is usually female. There may be associated sexual assault. Examination of the scene may reveal a ligature either in situ or near the body. The absence of the ligature is a pointer towards homicide. Examination of the neck with a magnifying lens may reveal fibres.

Artefacts

Ligature marks are occasionally mimicked by normal skin creases or by, for example, cracks caused by fires (Fig. 130). Putrefaction may accentuate skin creases or may cause the neck to expand against neck jewellery.

Throttling

Homicidal strangulation using the hands applies great pressure to localized areas (Fig. 131). Extensive fractures of the hyoid bone or of the laryngeal cartilages may be found with associated, but localized, bruising of the strap muscles of the neck. Such fractures tend to occur in older subjects, where the cartilaginous structures of the larynx are often ossified and brittle.

External findings on the neck in throttling include bruises produced by the digits and scratches caused by the nails.

Throttling may be accidental in sexual intercourse but usually it is a homicidal act.

Mechanism of death

In general, compression of the neck can apply pressure to the airway, to the jugular veins, to the carotid arteries or sinuses or to nerves. Pressure on the baroreceptors of the carotid sinus, the carotid sheaths and the carotid body may be followed by reflex cardiac arrest such that the deceased shows facial pallor rather than cyanosis or petechiae.

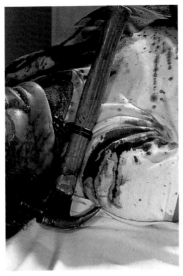

Fig. 129 Suicidal strangulation by ligature (putrefied).

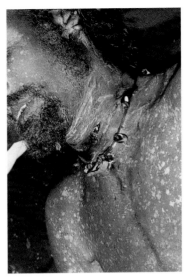

Fig. 130 Neck cracks in fire death.

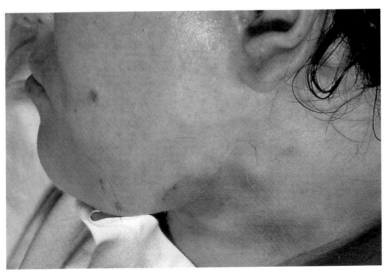

Fig. 131 Throttling injuries.

16 / Drowning

Drowning may be accidental (majority), suicidal or homicidal. Alcohol abuse is an important factor in accidental drowning and toxicology is an important component of the investigation of drowning.

Dry drowning

The clinical history suggests entry into water but the autopsy reveals no evidence of water inhalation into the lungs. The mechanism of death may be a vagally mediated cardiac arrest following contact of water with the laryngeal inlet.

Wet drowning

In wet drowning, there are signs of water inhalation into the lungs. The signs may be subtle or very obvious and include:

- *Froth in the airways.* The froth may emerge from the mouth as a plume (Fig. 132).
- *Overinflation of the lungs.* Peripheral displacement of air by water distends the air spaces and the medial aspects of each lung approach the midline. The lateral aspects of the visceral pleurae may show rib markings.

The heavy head and the limbs may be abraded by objects on the bottom, particularly in fast-flowing waters. Crabs often cause post-mortem damage, especially around the eyes and ears. Such artefacts need to be distinguished from bona fide ante-mortem injury.

In homicide, weights are sometimes employed to try to keep a body immersed. The limbs may also be bound (Fig. 133).

Diatoms. Diatoms are tiny plants and are ubiquitous in nature (Fig. 134). The presence of similar diatoms in the bone marrow of the deceased and in a sample of the inhaled water may infrequently help to establish the diagnosis of drowning.

Death in the bath

Four questions should spring to mind for the case of a female found drowned in a bath:

- Is it homicide?
- Is it a drug overdose?
- Is she an epileptic?
- Is the death a complication of pregnancy?

Suicidal immersion in the bath is not uncommon for both sexes. Occasionally, the deceased may have used a simple lever system, such as a block of wood across the bath, to prevent flotation.

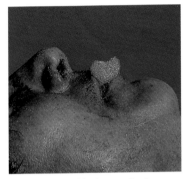

Fig. 132 Plume of froth emerging from mouth.

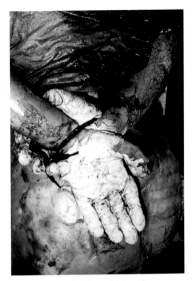

Fig. 133 Bound wrists with 'washer-woman' changes to skin of hands.

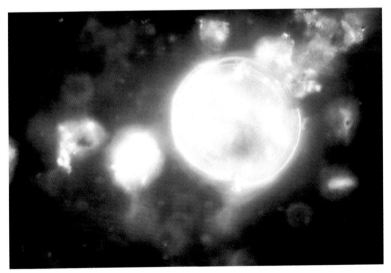

Fig. 134 Diatoms.

17 / **Diving deaths**

Diving involves the use of snorkelling equipment or self-contained underwater breathing apparatus (scuba) gear. Most deaths associated with diving are caused by drowning, though dysbaric problems may have caused or contributed to the drowning. Dysbarism and barotrauma are unlikely to occur in snorkellers.

Natural disease may also cause the death, particularly in older divers. Occasionally, the body of the diver is not recovered although equipment may be found. Borrowed equipment may cause identification problems. Infrequently, a wet suit is recovered which shows evidence of shark attack (Fig. 135).

Post-mortem examination

The pathologist may find it useful to have an expert adviser present at the autopsy, especially if that person has a detailed knowledge of the diving apparatus and is able to examine it.

Key points

- Consideration of the circumstances of death—should special examination, such as CAT scan or X-ray, be performed before autopsy?
- External examination:
    - especially for evidence of trauma
    - crepitus of the skin should be tested for
    - an otoscope may reveal ruptured eardrums.
- Removal of brain with clamping of arterial supply:
    - bubbles should be looked for on release of the clamps under water (Fig. 136)
    - the brain is retained for neuropathological examination.
- The chest should be examined for pneumothorax.
- The heart is also examined for gas bubbles. Froth in the chambers is readily apparent if in sufficient volume to have caused death.
- The heart should also be examined for congenital problems such as patent foramen ovale. Recent research has indicated that connections between systemic and pulmonary circulations are important to the development of decompression illness.
- A comprehensive collection of tissues should be sampled for histology.
- Putrefaction renders a search for gas bubbles invalid.
- Full toxicology is recommended.

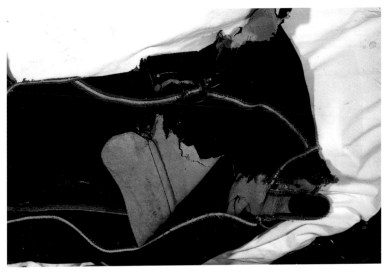

Fig. 135 Shark teeth marks on wet suit.

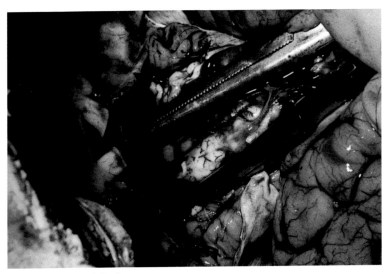

Fig. 136 Air bubbles in basilar artery.

18 / Autoerotic death

Definition This term is applied to accidental deaths that occur during individual, usually solitary, sexual activity in which some type of apparatus, used to enhance the sexual stimulation, causes unintended death. Autoerotic asphyxial death is the most common type but there are many variations (Fig. 137).

Aqua-eroticism. Aqua-eroticism is one of the more rare forms of autoerotic entertainment and employs near-drowning as the hypoxic stimulus. Cases present as drowning and there is evidence of previous unusual underwater activity.

Autoerotic asphyxia. In autoerotic asphyxial death, hanging is the usual cause of the accidental death. There may be padding or lubrication of the hanging device.

General features Autoerotic death has been described in males of varying ages but males between the ages of 15 and 25 are most at risk. Rare cases occur in females and such cases initially may be thought to be homicides, especially when the female is found dead and naked with only a ligature in situ.

Photographs or scrapbooks found at the scene may provide evidence of previous similar activity. Sexual literature, mirrors, sex aids and electrical sex toys or devices may also be found at the scene. These items may be absent in female autoerotic death although intra-vaginal foreign bodies or vibrators may be found.

Accidental electrocution may occur during autoerotic practice and there have been reports of items such as a toy train transformer, a motorized rotisserie and a television set being used in such practice. Investigators should be wary of potential electrocution.

Leather (Fig. 138), rubber and female underclothing are regular features in male autoerotic death. It is important to ascertain that bondage equipment could have been potentially released by the deceased.

Certain cases can be extremely bizarre, involving the use of cars, dental chairs, saddles, ski boots, tractors, hydraulic lifts, and a vast range of other paraphernalia. Typically, there is no history of depression and the deceased may be reported as being happily married. Suicide notes are absent.

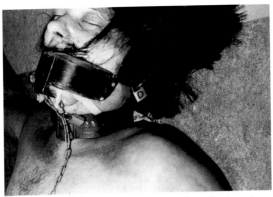

Fig. 137 Autoerotic asphyxia; note chains, wig, padlocks and bondage gear.

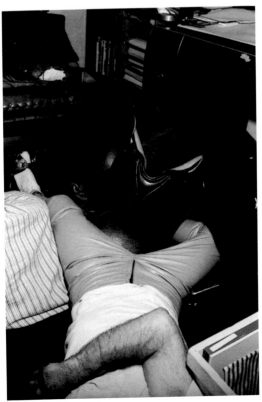

Fig. 138 Leather fetishism.

Homicide   Autoerotic activity is occasionally conducted by homosexual males acting in pairs as a way of protecting against accidental death. If death occurs, the possibility of a homicide should be considered.

Cases of homicide being modified to look like autoerotic deaths are described.

Injuries   Injuries are frequently absent because of protective devices or lubricant materials. Minor abrasions may be found; Figure 139 shows chafing marks left by a leather bondage strap (Fig. 140). Note the rubber pad which had separated the strap from the anal region.

Masturbation with a vacuum cleaner hose or a hair drier may sometimes cause injuries to the penis but such injuries are rare in fatal cases. In one of our cases, abrasions of a minor nature were noted at the base of the penis. In a case from Western Australia, there were no injuries to the penis but the underpants were impacted in the hose of the vacuum cleaner.

Fruit and vegetables   Fruit and vegetables are rarely used in autoerotic activity, but a case report from Western Australia describes fatal autoerotic asphyxia caused by a zucchini. This foreign body was impacted in the upper airway and it appeared likely that the deceased was using the zucchini to simulate fellatio. In a case complicated by faecal peritonitis, we found a 23-cm-long carrot, inserted per rectum, which had perforated the sigmoid colon.

Custom-built devices   Figure 141 shows an example of a total body autoerotic entrapment device. Such devices, indeed all the bondage magazines, sex aids and other equipment related to the death, may be removed by embarrassed relatives prior to reporting the death to the authorities.

Toxicology   Toxicology may reveal evidence of inhalation of volatiles; the male pictured in Figure 138 (p. 84) had been inhaling ether prior to falling off the saddle. Alcohol and other drugs may be identified but their use in autoerotic practice is rather uncommon, in our experience.

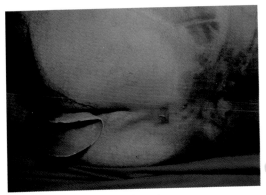

Fig. 139 Rubber pad between buttocks.

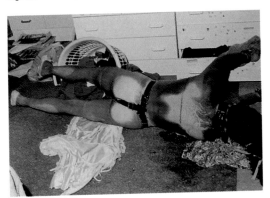

Fig. 140 Leather bondage straps.

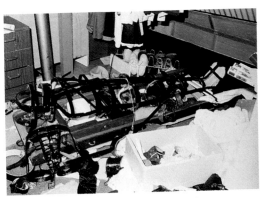

Fig. 141 Total body autoerotic entrapment device.

19 / **Sex**

Sexual offences

In sexual offences, the post-mortem examination is concerned not just with injuries to the genital tract but the injuries sustained elsewhere on the body. Rape is sometimes followed by homicide.

Genital examination

The genital tract is conveniently examined with adjacent areas such as perineum and anus. In the female, wounds are described according to site and the hymenal orifice dimensions measured, if relevant. Tears (lacerations), abrasions and bruises (Fig. 142) are typical injuries but, infrequently, slash or stab wounds are encountered (Fig. 143). Findings may include redness or oedema of the clitoris, irregularities of the hymen, if present, splits in the posterior fourchette and perineal or perianal bruising. Perianal or perivulval warts or condylomata may be encountered. The examination is done, not just to detail the injuries, but to provide specimens for forensic biology and microbiology. The distensibility of the vagina should be assessed digitally after taking specimens.

Investigations

Swabs. Swabs of vagina, cervix, anus and mouth for detection of semen or blood are collected. Such specimens are valuable for DNA studies. A blood sample is taken from the deceased for reference purposes.

Microbiology. Plain dry cotton wool swabs are also used to provide specimens for microbiological culture. Sexually transmitted disease is not uncommon and may form an important evidential link between victim and perpetrator. Stewarts transport medium is employed for the gonococcus swab and a smear should be made as well.

Photography. Injuries to sexual organs, the inner thighs and the perineum are photographed as part of the overall photographic record of the autopsy.

Foreign debris. Materials such as hairs, stains and fibres are collected. Adhesive tape may be employed to harvest foreign hairs from the pubic area. Occasionally, a foreign body is found within the vagina or anus (Fig. 144) as an incidental finding in an otherwise entirely natural death.

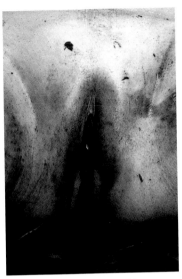

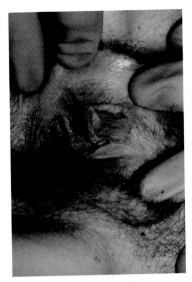

Fig. 142 Rape injuries in a child.

Fig. 143 Stab wounds to vagina.

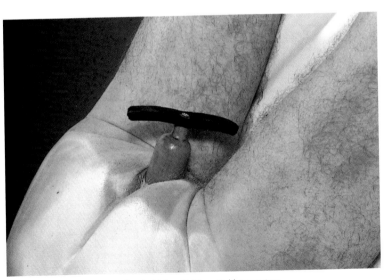

Fig. 144 Carved wooden phallus (with handle) inserted into rectum.

General investigations

A thorough overall inspection of the body is made for wounds, particularly bite marks (Figs 145 & 146) and defence injuries. The hands may carry evidence from an attacker and it may be useful to provide:

- nail clippings
- nail scrapings
- hand washings

for the forensic scientists. Bite marks can also be swabbed for traces of saliva.

Rape is occasionally accompanied by ritual acts involving sexually significant areas (Fig. 147). Figure 148 is a Polaroid print taken at the scene. It shows faecal stained impressions left by a broom handle which had been inserted into the rectum. All wounds should be photographed. Black and white, as well as colour photographs may be required for bite marks. A rule or other scale should be included in the photographs to aid subsequent interpretation.

Toxic shock syndrome

Toxic shock syndrome is a rare condition, diagnosed on the basis of strict clinical criteria rather than on pathological grounds.

Clinical criteria

1. Hypotension
2. Fever
3. Rash, typically a macular eruption
4. Desquamation of the rash, 1–2 weeks later
5. Multiple system failure.

Features

The syndrome has been linked to high-absorbency tampon use but it may accompany any source of the toxin, which is usually produced by certain strains of *Staphylococcus aureus*.

Pathologists should be wary of diagnosing toxic shock syndrome merely on the basis of finding a tampon at autopsy. Occasionally, especially in women in the early reproductive years, post-mortem autolysis of the uterus may lead the unwary to think of purulent exudate. In toxic shock syndrome associated with tampon use, there may be ulcers of upper vagina and cervix. A high vaginal swab is a useful investigation to identify any toxin-producing bacteria.

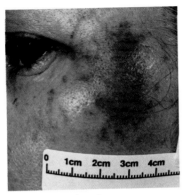

Fig. 145 Bite mark on face.

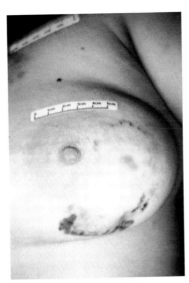

Fig. 146 Bite mark on breast (same case as Fig. 148).

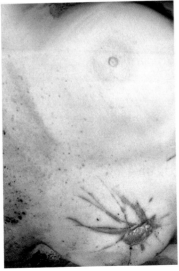

Fig. 147 Knife mutilation of one silicone breast and faint bite mark to the other.

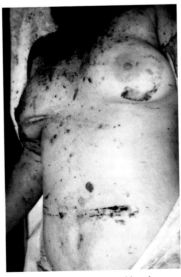

Fig. 148 Faecal smearing and beating.

Penile injuries

Mutilation

Penile injuries are not necessarily an indication of genital mutilation. There may be an innocent explanation such as sudden death in the lavatory and trapping of the penis between lavatory seat and the body as the body falls. Carnivore predation, particularly by cats and dogs (Fig. 149), is not uncommon in the domestic environment, the death typically occurring in a single person home.

Penile injury is occasionally encountered as a complication of autoerotic death, for example when an electrical device has been used for penile stimulation.

General features

Unusual marks are frequently found on the penis and include tattoos (Fig. 150), bite marks, love bites, vitiligo and numerous other lesions. Ticklers (Fig. 151) are subcutaneous brightly coloured adornments for the penis, intended to enhance sexual satisfaction. In some areas of the world, stones are inserted into the penile skin for similar purposes and also for initiation and religious significance.

Figure 152 shows a particularly striking example of vitiligo of the glans on the penis of an HIV-positive, hepatitis-B-positive, syphilitic homosexual who had been murdered. Such unusual features are occasionally helpful for purposes of identification.

The occurrence of spermatozoa at the penile meatus is not necessarily caused by ante-mortem ejaculation. Emission of semen is common in hangings or violent deaths.

Sexually transmitted disease

Venereal warts may be an indication of other sexually transmitted diseases. Investigation of such diseases may reveal a link between a homicide victim and a perpetrator. The classic diseases detected by taking vaginal or anal swabs include syphilis, gonorrhoea and lymphogranuloma venereum. Anal swabs may also reveal sexually transmitted salmonellosis, shigellosis or campylobacter. Protozoan diseases such as giardiasis and viral diseases such as herpes simplex may also be transmitted as a result of anal intercourse.

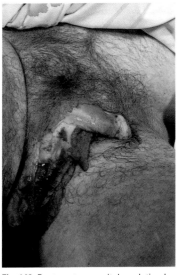

Fig. 149 Post-mortem genital predation by dog.

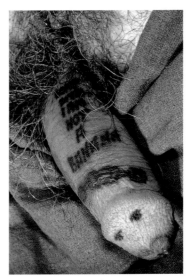

Fig. 150 Tattoo on penis.

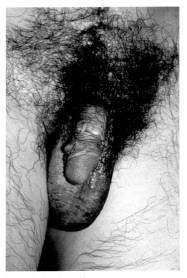

Fig. 151 Penile ticklers.

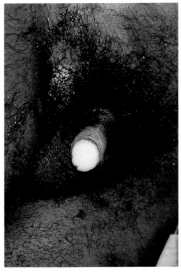

Fig. 152 Vitiligo of penile glans.

The human immunodeficiency virus (HIV) may be transmitted sexually or by contact with infected blood. About one-third of those infected develop symptoms in the early phase, often a fever with or without enlarged lymph nodes and a rash. There then follows a prolonged symptom-free stage. Most infected individuals advance to full-blown acquired immunodeficiency syndrome (AIDS) within 10 years but the range of time required to develop AIDS may be between 2 and 15 years. The immune devastation caused by the HIV virus is a direct consequence of its evolution in the body. The viral level rises gradually in parallel with a decline in the T helper lymphocyte population.

The forensic pathologist considers all bodies to be potentially infective. Testing for HIV antibodies in our institution is limited to those bodies where consideration of the circumstances of death suggests that HIV positivity is likely. These circumstances may also suggest the possibility of hepatitis viruses and other infections potentially hazardous to the pathologist.

Body fluids Body fluids considered to transmit HIV include blood, semen, vaginal secretions, and cerebrospinal, peritoneal, amniotic, pericardial and synovial fluids. Other fluids are not implicated in the transmission of HIV unless they contain visible blood.

Features Sudden death in HIV infection is becoming increasingly recognized, especially in persons who have kept their infection secret. A knowledge of the huge range of clinical features demonstrated in HIV and AIDS may alert the pathologist to the diagnosis. In those people newly diagnosed as being HIV-positive, suicides have occurred where counselling services have been absent.

About 10% of patients with AIDS present because of neurological symptoms, but up to three-quarters of them will have evidence of neurological disease. This disease may be caused by a cryptococcal infection of the brain (Fig. 153), by a direct effect of HIV on the brain or from other infective causes such as toxoplasmosis (Fig. 154).

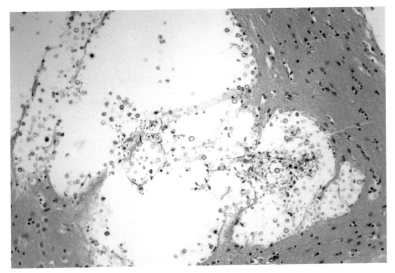

Fig. 153 Cryptococcus in brain.

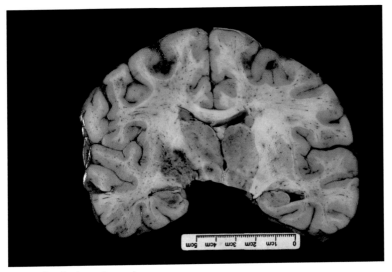

Fig. 154 Cerebral toxoplasmosis.

Common terminal infections in HIV/AIDS

Cryptococcosis

Cryptococcus neoformans is a fungus found in soil and in bird droppings, particularly droppings from pigeons. It is a yeast cell with a thick mucoid capsule which is classically demonstrable in tissue sections using Indian ink to form a dark background against which the capsules are clearly seen.

The fungus may be inhaled, initiating a mucoid pneumonia prior to dissemination by the blood. Cryptococcus has a particular affinity for the meninges, where it causes a gelatinous meningitis. Such brains tend to be very slippery when handled at post-mortem examination although the meningitis itself is very difficult to see macroscopically.

The organisms may form collections within the parenchyma, often with little or no inflammatory response. These collections macroscopically look like 'puddles of mucus' or 'gelatinous pseudocysts'. Histological examination shows the organisms within mucoid pools (Fig. 153, p. 94).

Cryptococcosis is believed to be the commonest type of cerebral mycosis in AIDS sufferers.

Toxoplasmosis

Toxoplasma gondii is a protozoan infecting cats and other animals. Food contaminated with feline faeces may cause transmission to humans. Toxoplasma encephalitis is a common complication in HIV infection and the organism is a common cause of intracerebral mass lesions (Fig. 154, p. 94). In toxoplasmosis, there is dissemination of organisms throughout the tissues. There may be a toxoplasma myocarditis (Fig. 155) which is clinically silent compared to those neurological manifestations of the disease. Figure 156 shows a Giemsa-stained preparation of toxoplasma within the brain. The diagnosis is confirmed by serology.

Pneumocystosis

Pneumocystis carinii is currently believed to be a fungus rather than a protozoan. In the developed countries, pneumocystis pneumonia is the commonest cause of death of HIV-infected people. The pneumonia is macroscopically similar to pancreatic tissue and is thus described as pancreatization. The organisms grow slowly in the alveoli of the lungs in association with exudates, the appearance being highlighted by silver stains (Fig. 157).

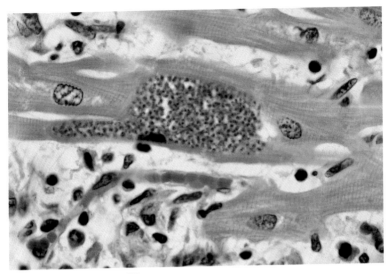

Fig. 155 Toxoplasma myocarditis.

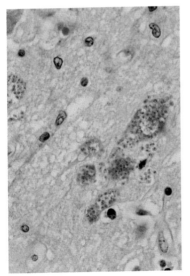

Fig. 156 Toxoplasma encephalitis.

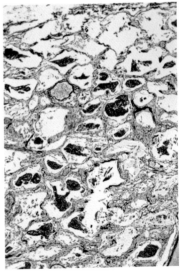

Fig. 157 Pneumocystis pneumonia.

21 / **Fire**

Fire may be used occasionally to try to mask a homicide. The majority of fire deaths, however, are usually accidents or suicide. Burns due to dry heat may demonstrate a wide variety of appearances depending on:

* temperature
* time
* fuel content of the body
* protective coverings, for example clothes.

Surface burns

Burns can be assessed using three degrees according to the severity of depth of tissue damage. The area burnt may be calculated using the 'rule of nines'. These terms are comprehensively explained in many textbooks of medicine.

A third degree burn is the most serious and extends to fat, muscle and bone.

Scalds

A scald (Fig. 158) is tissue damage caused by hot liquid, the most common source of such a liquid being the kettle or the bath. Scalds from a hot tap may typically cause a dripping pattern of scalding down the body. There may be a horizontal pattern to the scald if there has been immersion in hot liquid. Scalds are bright red when fresh and can be mimicked by iatrogenic problems, such as leakage of an irritant intravenous injection into the tissues (Fig. 159).

Incineration

The heat generated by fire may cause artefacts resembling evidence of violence. Commonly, there are:

* splits (Fig. 160)
* amputations
* heat haematomas.

The 'pugilistic' attitude of the body may cause alarm to the uninitiated (Fig. 161).

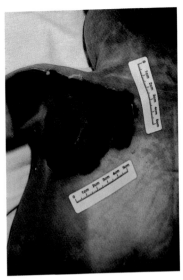

Fig. 158 Scald.

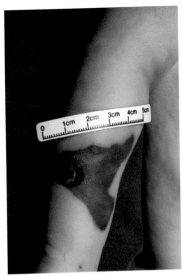

Fig. 159 Complication of an injection mimicking a scald.

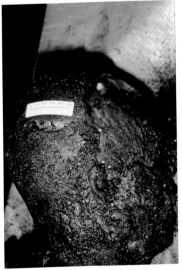

Fig. 160 Heat-related split in skin.

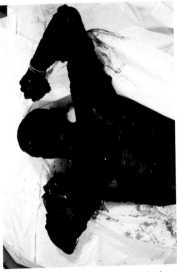

Fig. 161 Pugilistic attitude of burnt body.

Post-mortem findings Death may have resulted acutely from the inhalation of carbon monoxide and/or toxic fumes rather than from the effects of burning. In burnt or scalded patients who have survived for some days, infection may be the cause of death. Important points for the autopsy include:

- Orientation of the body. There may be severe distortion of body cavities and planes caused by fire and it is important to establish the correct anatomy prior to dissection.
- Exclusion of ante-mortem injuries. Self-mutilation may be occasionally found in a burnt body (Fig. 162) and may be indicative of a psychiatric illness or the consequences of drug abuse.
- Examination of the airways for heat damage and soot deposition, particularly the trachea and main bronchi. The tissues may also show a pinkness due to carboxyhaemoglobin.
- There may also be evidence of swallowing of burnt debris, with soot deposition in oesophagus and stomach.
- Toxicological specimens for carbon monoxide, cyanide and other toxic substances. It is important to screen for alcohol and drugs. Blood cultures under sterile conditions should be taken if there is a possibility of septicaemia.
- Full histology. Evidence of inhalation of soot (Fig. 163) suggests that the deceased was alive when the fire started. Natural disease may be a reason for failure to escape from the fire. Artefacts caused by heat may imitate disease and one example is the spurious thickening of pulmonary blood vessels (mimicking pulmonary hypertension) in heat-altered lung (Fig. 164).

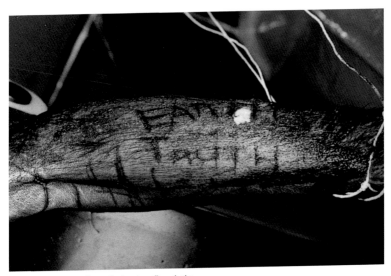

Fig. 162 Recent self-mutilation in a fire victim.

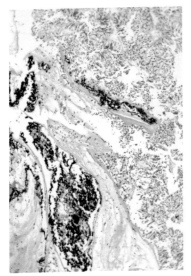

Fig. 163 Soot in airway.

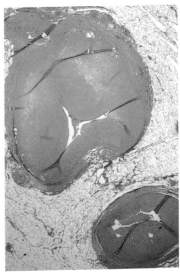

Fig. 164 Artefactual thickening of pulmonary blood vessels in heat-altered lung.

Identification of the fire victim

Fires may be very destructive and there may be little material available for identification of the deceased (Fig. 165). Occasionally, a metal prosthesis such as a plate in a long bone (Fig. 166) provides useful indication of identity. The most commonly employed method of confirmation of identification in fire victims involves the teeth but skeletal radiology is also widely used (see p. 15).

Dentition

The dentition survives incineration very well. However, at high temperatures, the enamel caps may separate from the remainder of the teeth, and an attempt should be made to recover these from the scene. The cheeks act as insulation and protect posterior teeth for a considerable time, but anterior teeth are far more vulnerable.

At retrieval, the teeth may be charred and friable (Fig. 167). Stabilization of the teeth and jaws with a glue that can later be dissolved away with a suitable solvent is recommended to ensure complete recovery in such cases, and to facilitate jaw removal. The jaws should ideally be removed in all cases of dental identification, but this is particularly important in the case of incineration. The dentition should always be documented photographically after removal of the jaws from the remains. The tongue is likely to be swollen, and may obscure the occlusal surfaces of posterior teeth. It should be carefully dissected away from these teeth before examination can be performed (Fig. 168).

Dental materials

Dental materials are susceptible to high temperatures in different ways. Silver amalgam loses mercury at around 100°C. At 500°C silver oxide is formed, which has a distinctive black powdery appearance. By around 1000°C the restoration has totally vaporized. Dental golds melt at temperatures above 850°C, and dental acrylics melt and ignite at 200–250°C. Metal denture bases survive temperatures of up to 1100°C. Semiprecious alloys may survive up to 1000°C.

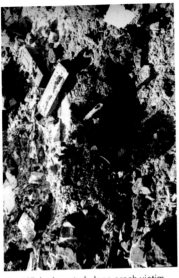

Fig. 165 Incinerated plane crash victim.

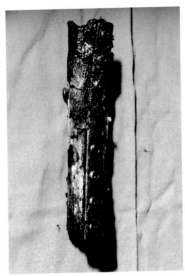

Fig. 166 Metal plate recovered from plane crash victim.

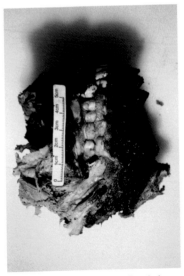

Fig. 167 Teeth removed from fire victim.

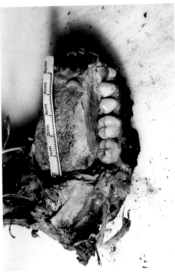

Fig. 168 Dissection of the tongue away from the posterior teeth.

22 / **Occupational disease**

In certain countries, there is legislation concerning compensation payable to the families of workers who are killed as a result of exposure to harmful chemicals or substances.

Pneumoconiosis

Pneumoconiosis is a general term describing lung disease consequent to the inhalation of dust.

Anthracosis

One of the commonest types of pneumoconiosis is anthracosis, caused by the inhalation of atmospheric soot particles or cigarette smoke. Anthracosis does not necessarily impair pulmonary functions but it does cause the blackened appearance seen commonly in adult lungs.

Asbestos-related disease

Asbestos is a generic term for naturally occurring fibrous silicates of magnesium. In contrast to the inhalation of atmospheric soot, inhalation of asbestos may cause significant pulmonary disease. Crocidolite (blue asbestos) is the most dangerous form.

Asbestos bodies. Inhaled asbestos fibres tend to become trapped in the respiratory bronchioles of the lower lobes of the lungs. They are subject to macrophage attack and become coated with protein and iron to form asbestos bodies. Asbestos bodies are one form of iron-coated or ferruginous bodies and they are conveniently demonstrated by the use of a Perls' stain (Fig. 169), which stains the iron.

Asbestosis. This term describes pulmonary fibrosis consequent upon asbestos exposure. Lungs so affected demonstrate a combination of fibrosis (Fig. 170) and occasional asbestos bodies. There may also be pleural plaques, often calcified, pleural effusions and pleural fibrosis. Lung carcinoma may develop as a complication of asbestosis, the most common type being adenocarcinoma.

Mesothelioma. Mesothelioma is a malignant neoplasm which tends to grow along pleural surfaces and into the lung tissues. This pleural malignancy causes diminution of the size of the lung by compression (Fig. 171). Mesothelioma is a complication of asbestos inhalation and asbestos bodies, but not necessarily asbestosis.

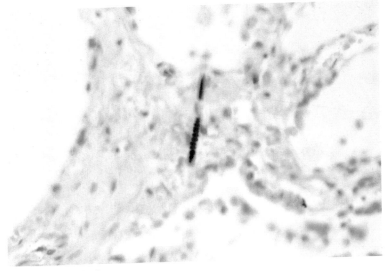

Fig. 169 Asbestos body.

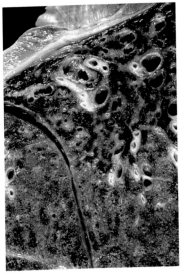

Fig. 170 Asbestosis.

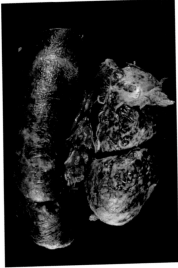

Fig. 171 Mesothelioma compressing one lung.

Silica-related disease

Silica dust is found wherever rock is fragmented. Miners and workers in the stone and slate industry are at risk of inhalation of silica.

Silicosis. Chronic silica inhalation produces silicosis, characterized by pulmonary fibrosis with silicotic nodules. The latter consist of birefringent silica crystals surrounded by concentric rings of fairly acellular fibrous tissue. Such crystals should not be confused with embolized foreign body material associated with intravenous drug abuse.

In any form of pneumoconiosis, the pulmonary fibrosis which develops is frequently complicated by pulmonary hypertension and cor pulmonale.

Silicate

Large areas of the world are planted with sugar cane and waste material, left over after harvesting, is sometimes burnt. Exposure to the dust and fumes from this activity commonly causes inhalation of silicate, which causes a reaction in the lungs similar to that of silica. The silicate crystals are also birefringent (Figs 172 & 173) but are usually more spicular and longer than silica crystals. The silicate material is seen not only in the lungs of the cane workers but also in the lungs of their families and neighbours.

Infections

Abattoir workers and those who work with animal products risk exposure to various hazards within the meat. Well-recognized bacterial problems are caused by the genus *Brucella*.

Q fever

In Queensland, Australia, there may be exposure to rickettsial infection such as Q fever. This disease is caused by *Coxiella burnetii*. The symptoms are abrupt and are similar to flu.

Cardiac inflammation is a rare but usually fatal complication. Figure 174 shows a Q fever myocarditis in a 21-year-old meat inspector. The liver demonstrates the fibrin-rich granuloma (Fig. 175) typical of the disease; an individual granuloma may contain a fat droplet.

Valvular disease may also develop as a consequence of Q fever.

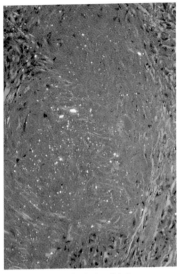

Fig. 172 Silicate (polarized) in lung.

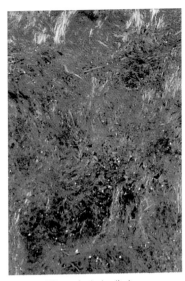

Fig. 173 Silicate (polarized) plus anthracotic pigment in hilar lymph node.

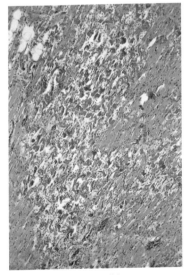

Fig. 174 Q fever myocarditis.

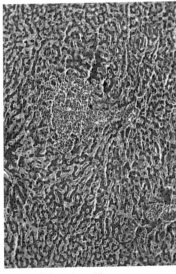

Fig. 175 Q fever hepatitis.

23 / Forensic neuropathology

Forensic neuropathology deals with the consequences of diseases and injuries affecting the central and peripheral nervous systems. It is an enormous subject and only certain facets of it will be discussed.

Dementia

Causes

There are multiple causes for dementia including infective causes such as neurosyphilis, chronic alcohol abuse, trauma and normal pressure hydrocephalus. There is marked impairment of higher mental functions, usually progressive. Alzheimer's disease and Pick's disease are two examples of primary dementias.

Alzheimer's disease. This disease is the most common primary dementia. The brain demonstrates atrophy, which is most marked in the temporal (Fig. 176) and frontal poles with compensatory hydrocephalus. Histology demonstrates neurofibrillary tangles, senile plaques containing amyloid and a widespread loss of neurones.

Pick's disease. This primary dementia has clinical signs similar to Alzheimer's disease and there is marked temporal and frontal pole atrophy, but Pick's disease can often be distinguished by the relative sparing of the posterior two-thirds of the first temporal gyrus. When severe, the gyri of the affected brain are so atrophic as to have a 'knife-edge' appearance (Fig. 177).

Punch-drunk syndrome. This syndrome is also described as dementia pugilistica. The syndrome has been recognized in boxers sustaining chronic head trauma over a number of years. The cerebral abnormalities include cerebral atrophy, Alzheimer-type neurofibrillary tangles (Fig. 178) without plaques and a torn, fenestrated or shrunken septum pellucidum.

Forensic significance

Dementia in one member of a household is a potential source of stress to the other family members, this stress occasionally being manifest as homicide.

Complications of dementia include problems in swallowing, accompanied by lung abscess or by aspiration pneumonia, and by a tendency to wander. These complications commonly bring the demented patients to their demise.

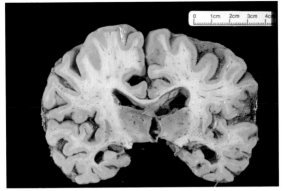

Fig. 176 Alzheimer's disease.

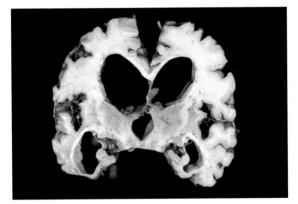

Fig. 177 Pick's disease.

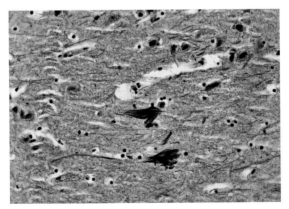

Fig. 178 Neurofibrillary tangles in dementia pugilistica.

Cerebral trauma

Blunt trauma to the head can produce a number of acute, subacute or chronic conditions, many of which are associated with brain damage.

Types of injury   ***Subgaleal haemorrhage.*** This is a collection of blood between the scalp and the skull (Fig. 179) and is seen most commonly in infants, often as a consequence of a road traffic accident. Skull fractures may be absent but, not uncommonly, the brain in fatal cases demonstrates cerebral oedema.

Extradural haematoma. This haematoma (Fig. 180) arises as a result of bleeding from a meningeal blood vessel, usually in association with a skull fracture. The haematoma pushes the dura (see diagram below) against the brain thus producing raised intracranial pressure.

Subarachnoid haemorrhage. Traumatic subarachnoid haemorrhage needs to be distinguished from that caused by rupture of an aneurysm (Fig. 181). Patchy subarachnoid haemorrhage, often combined with other forms of intracranial haemorrhage, is seen in a variety of head injuries. More diffuse examples may be seen following a blow to the side or the back of the neck, particularly in intoxicated individuals.

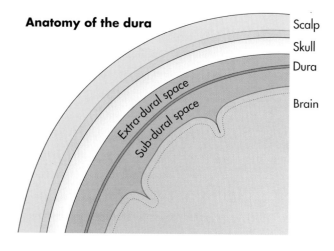

Anatomy of the dura

Scalp
Skull
Dura

Brain

Extra-dural space
Sub-dural space

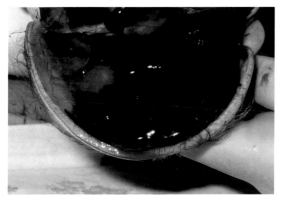

Fig. 179 Subgaleal haemorrhage.

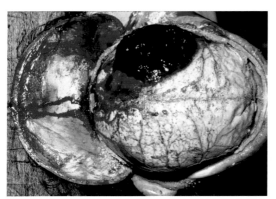

Fig. 180 Extradural haematoma.

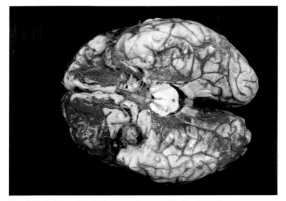

Fig. 181 Subarachnoid haemorrhage with display of aneurysm.

Types of injury
(contd)

Subdural haematoma. This is a very common complication of head injury. The dura is a tough membrane covering the brain and a haematoma between the dura and the brain is a subdural haematoma (Fig. 182), usually easily distinguished from the extradural haematoma.

A subdural haematoma may be accompanied by focal subarachnoid haemorrhage. In the solidified state, the haematoma can be weighed, the weight being a useful guide to pressure effects. In the liquid (fresh) state, the subdural haematoma over the top of the brain is distinguished from a subarachnoid haemorrhage by the fact that it washes off (Fig. 183). A subdural haematoma may occur with relatively trivial trauma particularly in alcoholics and the elderly where brain shrinkage and cerebral atrophy are predisposing factors.

It is usually possible to age a subacute or chronic subdural haematoma, using histological guidelines. The estimate of age may be relevant to an alleged previous assault.

Shaken baby
syndrome

Subdural haematoma is a feature of non-accidental injury in infants and children. There may be associated injury to spinal cord and to the eyes, these injuries being caused by shaking.

The injuries to the spinal cord may be subtle and usually consist of recent and/or old haemorrhage in the membranes.

Histological examination of an eye may reveal retinal haemorrhages in the shaken infant syndrome. Haemorrhages also occur in a subhyaloid position and in the choroid and sclera. Frequently these haemorrhages may coalesce. Retinal detachment is also a possibility.

Spinal cord
injury

Haematomyelia. This term describes contusions within the spinal cord (Fig. 184), usually arising as a consequence of extension or flexion injury to the spine. Rigidity of the spine, for example in cervical spondylosis or in ankylosing spondylitis, increases the risk of such injury. Haematomyelia is accompanied by oedema which may extend proximally, particularly in the cervical area, to cause respiratory arrest. The injury is seen infrequently as a complication of facial assault and may occur in isolation without any injury to the brain.

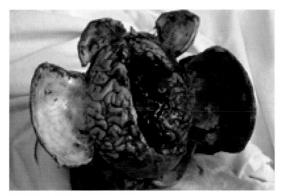

Fig. 182 Subdural haematoma.

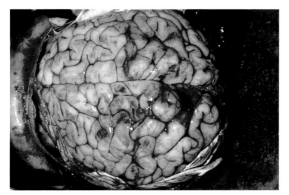

Fig. 183 Fresh subdural haematoma displaced to one side as dura removed.

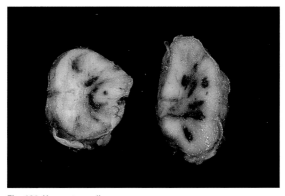

Fig. 184 Haematomyelia.

Coup and contrecoup

Contusions on the surface of the brain are characteristic of non-missile head injury. In contusional injury to the brain, the pia-arachnoid is not torn and, if it were, such an injury would be described as a cerebral laceration.

Coup contusion. This term describes bruising to the surface of the brain at the point of impact of blunt trauma. Surface contusions tend to occur at the crests of gyri. Fractures may be absent. Coup contusions are often more severe in relation to a blow to the stationary head than when the moving head is suddenly stopped.

If a person falls forward, striking the forehead on a hard surface, there may be an injury to the forehead and there may also be coup contusion (Fig. 185) or contusions to the front of the brain. There are unlikely to be any contusions to the back of the brain, for the reasons discussed below.

Contrecoup contusion. If a person falls on to the same hard surface, but this time striking the back of the head, there may be an injury to the scalp at the back of the head, often associated with a vertical hairline fracture, but there is unlikely to be any bruising to the back of the brain. There may be, however, bruising to the front of the brain and such bruising is described as a contrecoup contusion. This apparent paradox is explainable on the basis of:

- the shape and smoothness of the structures supporting the brain, particularly the skull
- the complex dynamics of brain movement inside the head.

In general, contusions to the surface of the brain are most commonly found on frontal and temporal poles. They provide evidence of head injury.

Contrecoup fracture. This relatively uncommon complication of contrecoup contusion may cause puzzlement. Typically, the thin orbital plates of the anterior cranial fossa may be fractured (Fig. 186) although the fall has been on to the back of the head. The shaved area of occipital scalp injury is shown in Figure 187, the injury showing a combination of laceration, abrasion and bruising.

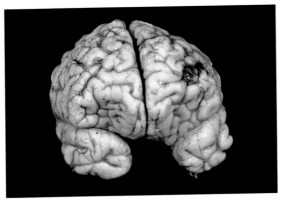

Fig. 185 Coup contusion to frontal area.

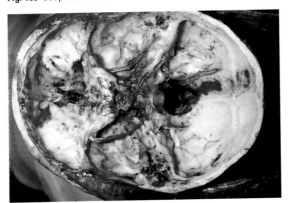

Fig. 186 Contrecoup fracture of orbital plate.

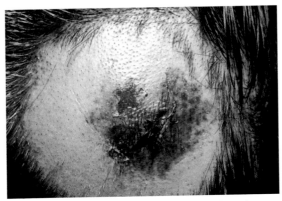

Fig. 187 Occipital scalp injury producing fractures shown in Figure 186.

Diffuse axonal injury

Diffuse axonal injury (DAI) has been briefly mentioned elsewhere (see p. 71). This severe brain injury is characterized clinically by the absence of any lucid interval and by persistence of an unconscious or vegetative state until death.

There are three distinct features to the neuropathology of diffuse axonal injury:

- *A lesion in the corpus callosum.* In most of the cases seen by forensic pathologists, the lesion is an area of haemorrhage. In cases where there is a long interval between injury and death, there may be a shrunken, cystic focus.
- *Lesions in the brain stem.* The appearance of these lesions is in parallel with the type of lesion seen in the corpus callosum. Typically, there are haemorrhages in the dorsolateral quadrant of the rostral brain stem, these haemorrhages often being small.
- *Diffuse damage to axons.* The damage is not visible macroscopically although its presence may be suggested by the occurrence of gliding contusions (Fig. 188). These contusions are defined as focal haemorrhages in the cerebral cortex and subjacent white matter at the superior margins of the cerebral hemispheres. Histological examination of the white matter shows swellings on nerve fibres, these swellings being known as retraction balls.

Odontoid peg dislocation

Features

The severe destruction caused by rheumatoid arthritis in the synovial joints of the upper cervical spine renders a patient at risk of odontoid peg dislocation during manipulation of the head. This manipulation may occur during the administration of anaesthesia or even during more mundane activity, such as having a bath (as in the case illustrated). Figure 189 shows the odontoid peg protruding into the foramen magnum while Figure 190 shows the resulting crush effect on the spinal medulla.

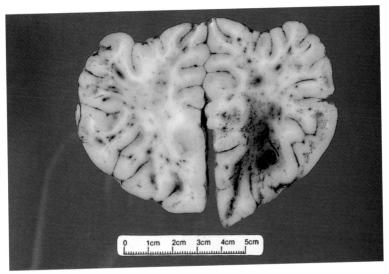

Fig. 188 Gliding contusions.

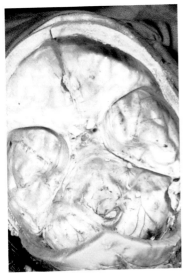

Fig. 189 Odontoid peg dislocation.

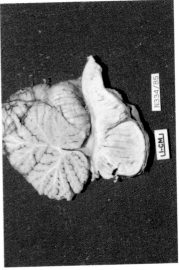

Fig. 190 Crushed spinal medulla.

Embolism and the brain

Brain embolism

Trauma to the head accompanied by disruption of the brain can, if the patient survives long enough, result in small amounts of brain entering the dural venous sinuses. The brain tissue is carried to the heart and is subsequently embolized throughout the body. Embolized brain is difficult to recognize in paraffin-embedded tissue; frozen section for fat may help with its localization.

Fat embolism to the brain

Fat embolism is a concern whenever a patient has fractures, trauma to subcutaneous tissues and in a variety of other situations. When fat is released into the circulation, it consists of small, deformable globules and many of them are removed by the lungs before they reach the brain. In cases of fulminant fat embolism to the brain, the brain may appear macroscopically normal on coronal section but if survival is longer than a few days, the white matter becomes diffusely studded with petechial haemorrhages (Fig. 191). This appearance is not pathognomonic of fat embolism but is also seen in disseminated intravascular coagulation and in hypoxic brain damage.

The white matter petechial haemorrhages are described as being of ring and ball type, because of their pericapillary distribution (Fig. 192). The fat can be demonstrated by frozen section of brain and oil red O staining (Fig. 193).

Hypoxic brain damage

Features

The brain requires a constant supply of oxygen and any diminution in that supply can cause a number of cerebral lesions.

Hypotension. An abrupt fall in blood pressure followed by a return to normal may cause boundary zone ischaemic damage. The boundary or watershed zones are areas of brain between the main arterial territories.

Cardiac arrest. Sustained cardiac arrest causes selective neuronal necrosis, most prominent in the hippocampus, and in certain layers of the cerebral cortex, certain basal nuclei and in Purkinje cells.

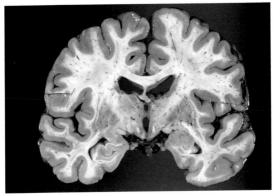

Fig. 191 Fat embolism to brain.

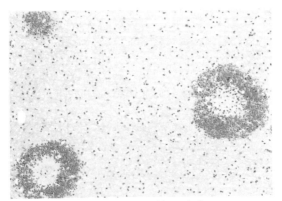

Fig. 192 Microscopic appearance of fat embolism.

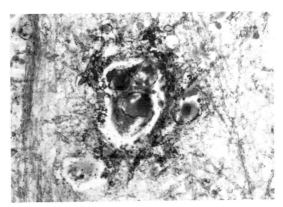

Fig. 193 Frozen section for fat.

Epilepsy

Cause Head injury is an important cause of epilepsy. Epilepsy may also arise as a complication of disease of the central nervous system and two of these diseases are considered.

Multiple sclerosis. Multiple sclerosis usually presents as recurrent attacks of neurological dysfunction. Such attacks may remit and recur randomly over many years.

In multiple sclerosis, lesions in the grey matter are generally regarded as a prerequisite for epilepsy to occur. Multiple sclerosis may present with epilepsy. The lesions consist of plaques of demyelination, these plaques often being scattered irregularly around the ventricles (Fig. 194).

Hydrocephalus. Hydrocephalus is most commonly caused by obstruction to the free flow of cerebrospinal fluid. The increase in the amount of fluid inside the brain produces a reduction in the amount of cerebral white matter, unless the obstruction is relieved by surgery. A consequence of neurosurgical intervention is fibrous scarring, a potent cause of epilepsy. Figure 195 shows a rare example of hydrocephalus caused by gliosis of the aqueduct. The patient died of status epilepticus.

Consequences Status epilepticus may be followed by acute selective neuronal necrosis of the hippocampus. In the majority of brains from epileptics, however, the histological abnormality, if present, is scarring of the hippocampus (hippocampal sclerosis). Occasionally, there is accompanying neuronal damage in cerebral cortex, certain basal nuclei and to Purkinje cells.

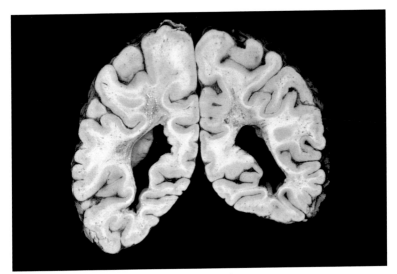

Fig. 194 Multiple sclerosis. Note the periventricular plaques.

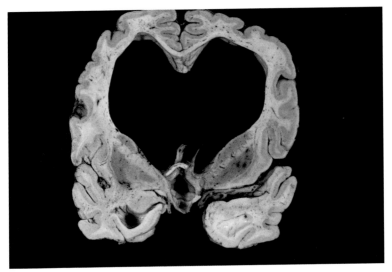

Fig. 195 Hydrocephalus.

24 / Alcohol

Definition   Ethyl alcohol or ethanol is the intoxicating product of fermentation in alcoholic drinks. The depressant effect of ethanol, commonly referred to as alcohol, may lead to reckless or self-destructive activity, manifest as accidents, suicides or homicides.

Sampling   The forensic pathologist should routinely take blood and urine for alcohol estimation in the following types of cases:

- homicides
- accidents: sampling of blood and urine for alcohol analysis is particularly pertinent to fires, drowning, occupational trauma and transportation fatalities—in the absence of blood or urine, bile or vitreous humour may be used instead
- suicide
- certain natural diseases
- chronic alcoholism.

Complications of alcohol abuse

Associations   There is a wide spectrum of disease associated with alcohol abuse. In fatalities, there may be effects of acute alcohol intoxication superimposed upon disease processes which have evolved as a result of chronic alcoholic abuse. The more common consequences of alcohol abuse on certain systems will be described.

These consequences of alcohol abuse are often very difficult to recognize in putrefied tissues (Figs 196 & 197). The chronic alcoholic may well live alone, having few visitors, and thus is at risk of unwitnessed death followed by putrefaction. Certain of the problems created by putrefaction will be discussed below, these problems applying not just to deaths in alcoholics.

Pancreas   Acute or chronic pancreatitis (Fig. 198) may occur and these conditions can be complicated by pseudocysts, chemical peritonitis, fat necrosis or diabetes. The dehydrating effect of alcohol and also a tendency for lactic acidosis to occur at high blood alcohol levels may fatally impair blood sugar levels.

Vitreous humour and post-mortem blood can be used for glucose estimation in a fresh corpse. A high vitreous glucose excludes hypoglycaemia but the reverse is not the case.

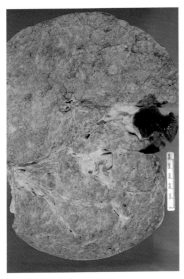

Fig. 196 Alcoholic cirrhosis.

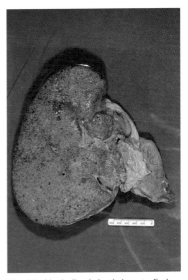

Fig. 197 Alcoholic cirrhosis in putrefied liver.

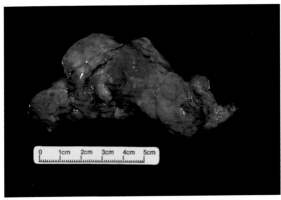

Fig. 198 Chronic pancreatitis.

Stomach   Acute or chronic gastritis is occasionally complicated by peptic ulcer or gastric haemorrhage. Mallory–Weiss tears occur at the gastro-oesophageal junction, usually as a sequel to vomiting, and are also associated with gastric haemorrhage. The hypovolaemia from gastric haemorrhage is frequently sufficient to produce heart failure, especially if there is an anaemia related to alcohol-associated dietary imbalance and nutritional deficiencies.

Liver   Fatty liver, alcoholic hepatitis and micronodular cirrhosis (Fig. 199) are all well-recognized complications of alcohol abuse. The fibrotic nature of cirrhosis means that connective tissue stains can be usefully employed when looking at the histology of putrefied liver. There may be oesophageal and sometimes gastric varices associated with the cirrhosis. Oesophageal varices may appear more prominent early in putrefaction (Fig. 200), but as putrefaction advances, lesions in the walls of the gastrointestinal tract become harder to diagnose.

    Conversely, it is also the case that putrefaction can mimic the effects of alcohol on the gastrointestinal tract and the pathologist should be wary of reading too much into the colours and texture of putrefied tissues.

    An important complication of alcoholic liver disease is a bleeding diathesis.

Lungs   The chronic alcoholic is frequently poor, malnourished and possibly immunocompromised because of cirrhosis. Infective disease, particularly tuberculosis, is a potential autopsy finding and the pathologist is required to take steps to prevent the spread of such infection. Tuberculosis of the lungs has a range of appearances but requires to be excluded if there is any evidence of caseation (Fig. 201).

Heart   Alcohol consumption of more than 5 units (50 g) daily is associated with increased risk of ischaemic heart disease. There is also an association between alcohol abuse and cardiomyopathy. Cardiomyopathies are heart muscle diseases of unknown cause and the most frequent type seen in alcoholics is the dilated or congestive cardiomyopathy, characterized by dilatation of left or right ventricles, or both.

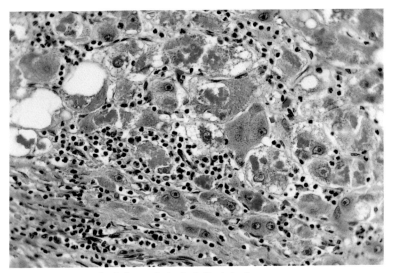

Fig. 199 Mallory's hyaline in liver cells in alcoholic cirrhosis.

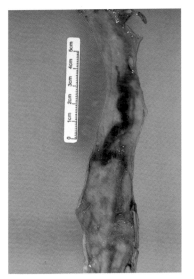

Fig. 200 Oesophageal varices in early putrefaction.

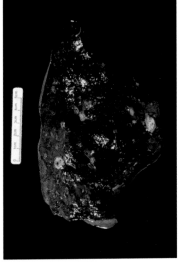

Fig. 201 Foci of caseous tuberculosis in lung of alcoholic male.

Heart (contd)

Putrefactive artefacts. Putrefaction creates artefactual dilatation of the chambers of the heart by virtue of gas formation, so dilated cardiomyopathy is difficult to diagnose with certainty under such circumstances. Putrefaction, however, should not increase the weight of the heart and this may be used as a more reliable guide.

Putrefaction also renders the macroscopic appearance of the myocardium poor for diagnosis of ischaemic heart disease. Connective tissue stains, however, may be usefully employed to examine the putrefied heart histologically (Fig. 202).

Cardiac changes associated with alcoholism may be subtle in the coronial context. The heart may not be enlarged and microscopic changes limited to focal interstitial fibrosis, myocyte hypertrophy and, occasionally, myo-intimal hyperplasia of small arteries (Fig. 203).

Brain

Direct toxic effects of alcohol include generalized cerebral atrophy and cerebellar superior vermal folial atrophy. Drinkers also have a tendency to fall, sustaining frontal or temporal contusions (Fig. 204) not uncommonly and also intracranial haemorrhage. Haemorrhages in the mamillary bodies and around the third ventricle may be seen in Wernicke–Korsakoff syndrome.

Acute intoxication

There is a wide spectrum of behaviour exhibited by different people at the same blood alcohol concentration, and hardened drinkers may tolerate blood alcohol concentrations that would be fatal in others.

In general, blood alcohol concentrations above 150–200 mg per 100 ml of blood in an occasional drinker are associated with demonstrable drunkenness which would be apparent to a sober observer. The reactions would be significantly impaired, such that self-defence to an assault might well be ineffectual.

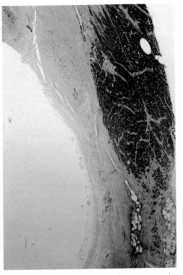

Fig. 202 Ischaemic fibrosis (green areas) in a putrefied myocardium.

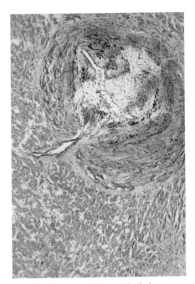

Fig. 203 Myo-intimal hyperplasia in cardiomyopathy.

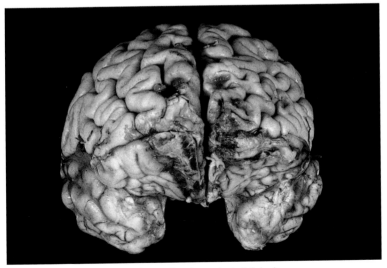

Fig. 204 Old frontal and temporal contusions in an alcoholic's brain.

25 / **Poisoning**

Definition Poisoning refers to the harmful effects of any substance when absorbed by the living body and may be accidental, suicidal or homicidal.

Features of poisoning Poisoning in children, especially young children, is usually accidental and typically involves household poisons. Such household poisons are occasionally used for suicide by older persons, but overdose of pharmaceutical drugs is more common.

Children under 2 years of age may be poisoned deliberately; such children are unlikely to open child-resistant containers or remove tablets from foil packs. Infrequently, deaths in such children are a complication of attempting to make a healthy child seem unwell (Munchausen syndrome by proxy).

The trends in suicidal poisoning in Australia have mirrored trends in the United Kingdom. In the 1970s, barbiturates were a favoured drug for overdose but over the past 15 years, cocktails of various antidepressants have been employed. Inhalation of exhaust gas (Fig. 205) has remained a common mode of suicide.

In exhaust gas poisoning, the pink coloration caused by carboxyhaemoglobin is very obvious in the vast majority of cases. This pink colour in the tissues is extremely slow to fade in fixative, so that a brain fixed in formal saline for 3 weeks retains its pink colour (Fig. 206).

Valuable clues to poisoning are often obtainable at the scene of death (Figs 207 & 208).

In homicidal poisoning, a problem of administration has to be overcome. How is an unusual taste to be disguised? How is an odd colour to be hidden? In one of our cases, the herbicide Paraquat, which is available as a brown liquid, was administered in a dish of prunes. There are rare cases describing the administration of poisons within resuscitative equipment such as intravenous lines and also the passing on of a lethal pill by a kiss.

One of the key requirements for a forensic pathologist is a high index of suspicion. Cases are occasionally encountered where there may appear to be one or several natural causes of death, yet analysis reveals evidence of drug overdose. Conversely, the post-mortem findings may be totally non-specific.

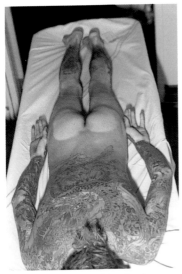

Fig. 205 Carbon monoxide poisoning.

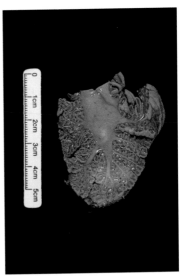

Fig. 206 Pink colour of carboxyhaemoglobin in fixed cerebellum.

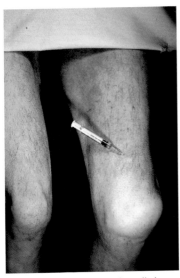

Fig. 207 Injection marks and needle in situ.

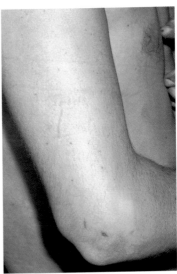

Fig. 208 Faint outline of tourniquet on skin of upper limb.

Safety Certain poisons, such as cyanide, are sometimes present in sufficient quantity in the stomach of the deceased to pose a risk to the pathologist. Some people have an inherited ability to smell cyanide but it is more appropriate to open the stomach within a safety cabinet rather than put staff at risk, when poisoning is suspected.

Pointers towards poisoning Pointers towards poisoning include:

- inconsistencies in the clinical history
- unusual or no employment
- a history of drug abuse or previous suicide attempt
- financial irregularities in the family/marital disharmony
- features noted on external examination of the body
- death not observed
- found dead and negative gross autopsy
- low self-esteem (Fig. 209).

External examination of the body may reveal an unusual smell, an unusual colour or an unusual mark. Powdery material on the lips or tablet residue in the mouth should be looked for.

On internal examination, there may be an unusual smell or unusual colour, especially in the gastrointestinal tract. A green bowel, for example, may be green because of copper salts (they may also produce a blue colour as in Fig. 210), dyes in the capsules of ingested pharmaceutical drugs (Fig. 211) or alternatively and perhaps more commonly, because of putrefaction. Patients in hospital are occasionally given innocuous dyes to monitor the transit time of the bowel contents and they may create an alarming appearance to the bowel wall. Intact tablets, pills or capsules are sometimes found in the stomach or small bowel and, infrequently, sufficient quantity of drug has been taken as to create a temporary 'bezoar' in the stomach.

In the majority of cases, no obvious tablet residue will be detected macroscopically in the stomach. An absence of empty medicine containers and/or a lack of a history of depression or other mental illness does not exclude a suicidal overdose.

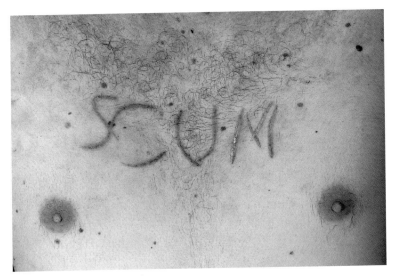

Fig. 209 Derogatory self-mutilation.

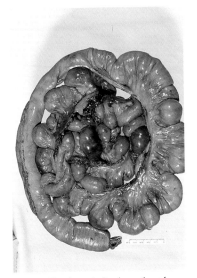

Fig. 210 Blue bowel after ingestion of copper oxychloride.

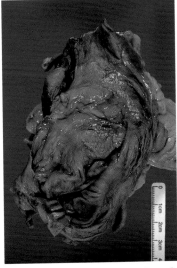

Fig. 211 Green caecum after overdose of green capsules.

Drug abuse

Intravenous drug abuse

A history of intravenous drug abuse is useful, but not always forthcoming, prior to autopsy. External features which may suggest this diagnosis include:

- injection marks (Fig. 207, p. 128) and damaged peripheral veins
- tattoos, especially examples that relate to the drug subculture
- emaciation and decreased personal hygiene
- occasionally, self-mutilation.

Complications

Intravenous drug abusers are subject to a huge range of complications but injection sites, lungs and heart are primarily involved by these complications.

Injection of material into a vein may lead to:

- poisoning by the active drug
- poisoning by a cutting agent
- introduction of microorganisms
- introduction of foreign bodies.

Narcotic poisoning may produce death extremely rapidly, even while the needle is still in the vein (Fig. 207, p. 128). Acute poisoning typically produces pronounced pulmonary oedema and congestion, a bloodstained plume of froth occasionally being seen emerging from the mouth.

The injection of foreign material may produce infection, including abscesses and thrombophlebitis, and a granulomatous reaction in and around the peripheral veins (Fig. 212). A similar reaction may be seen around pulmonary vessels, as a result of embolism (Fig. 213), and may result in chronic impairment of pulmonary function. Infection may manifest itself in the heart as tricuspid bacterial endocarditis.

Crushed tablets may be used for injection. Refractile particles, such as talc or cornstarch, evoke a variety of thrombotic and fibrotic lesions in the lung, lesions that may be absent with soluble fillers such as lactose or maltose. Refractile particles are usually easily identified in the lungs and peripheral injection sites by examining histological sections under polarized light (Figs 214 & 215).

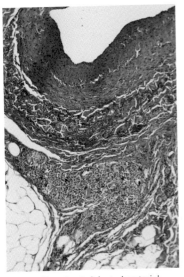

Fig. 212 Reaction to injected material around peripheral vein.

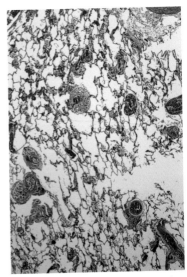

Fig. 213 Reaction to embolized injected material in lung.

Fig. 214 Polarization of crystalline material in Figure 212.

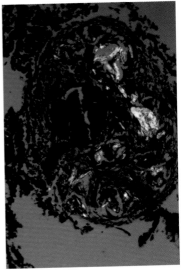

Fig. 215 Polarization of one of the granulomata seen in Figure 213.

Solvent abuse   A variety of organic solvents may be inhaled either for 'kicks' or to aid suicide. The term 'glue-sniffing' applies to the inhalation of toluene from glue, the glue usually poured into an empty crisp packet for ease of administration. Glue-sniffing is only one variant of solvent abuse; other variants, for example the inhalation of ether, are occasionally encountered in autoerotic asphyxia.

The most common cause of death appears to be sudden cardiac arrest, probably due to an arrhythmia. Another cause of death is inhalation of vomit.

At post-mortem examination, findings may be scant or absent. Occasionally there are petechial haemorrhages, skin lesions around the nares and a detectable odour on/in the body. The unfixed brain and an unsectioned lung, with the bronchus clamped off, are usually submitted for toxicological analysis along with the usual specimens of blood, urine and liver. Chronic solvent abusers may demonstrate mild fatty liver or a myocarditis on histological examination of their tissues.

In suicide, various devices may be utilized to inhale the solvent (Fig. 216).

Figures 217 and 218 show the source of propane inhalation for a death in custody. The middle-aged prisoner involved was found hanging. The usual victim of fatal solvent abuse is a teenager.

Amphetamines   Fatalities associated with the abuse of amphetamines and related drugs are not uncommon. A small proportion are due to the direct toxic effect of the drug but the greater proportion of deaths are due to injuries associated with motor vehicle accidents, homicide, suicidal hangings, multiple drug toxicity and stage jumping.

Para-methoxyamphetamine ('chicken yellow') is a designer drug derived from amphetamine and is the second most powerful hallucinogen after LSD. Methylene dioxymethyl amphetamine ('ecstasy') is taken at parties and at marathon dancing sessions. The users may be unaware of fatigue and the need for fluids. Dehydration may lead to cerebral haemorrhage and hyperthermic collapse. The autopsy may demonstrate scant findings.

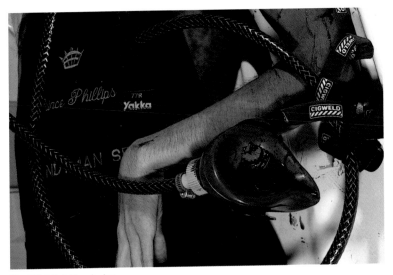

Fig. 216 Inhalation device.

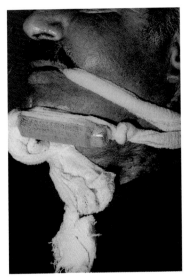

Fig. 217 Cigarette lighter within bandage used for hanging.

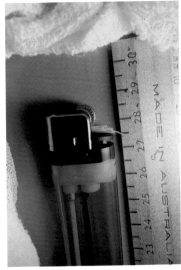

Fig. 218 Lighter wedged open with a match.

Heavy metals

All heavy metals have the capacity to interact with functional components of biological systems. This is an important characteristic of heavy metal poisoning. Some metals, such as copper, iron and zinc, play very important roles in the functioning of major enzyme systems, but become toxic at excessively high levels. Others, such as lead, arsenic, cadmium and mercury play no essential role in mammalian systems. These non-essential metals are of greatest general concern in human toxicology since exposure to them is relatively common.

Lead Lead poisoning may produce a blue line at the gingival margin (Fig. 219), especially when the dental hygiene is poor. Figure 220 shows an example of racial pigmentation of the gum for comparison.

Australia remains the world's largest producer of lead. Lead toxicology has been linked to changes in haemopoiesis, and neurological and renal function. Chronic exposure results in impaired cognitive development in children.

Arsenic One of the major uses of arsenic in the past was in cattle and sheep protection against tick infestation. Application was via dipping with arsenic-containing insecticides. In consequence, there are historically large numbers of such sites in rural and semi-rural areas of Australia where residents can be exposed to excessive concentrations of this metal which has a very long persistence in the environment. The commonest pathological changes observed as a result of chronic arsenic exposures include renal disease and skin lesions.

Cadmium Early studies of high cadmium exposure among occupationally exposed workers showed strong links with lung and renal malfunction and disease. Exposure to cadmium in the general environment has been linked with biochemical indicators of renal dysfunction.

Mercury Health effects from mercury exposure include kidney damage and neurological dysfunction.

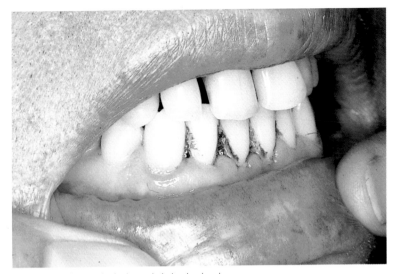

Fig. 219 Blue line at gingival margin in lead poisoning.

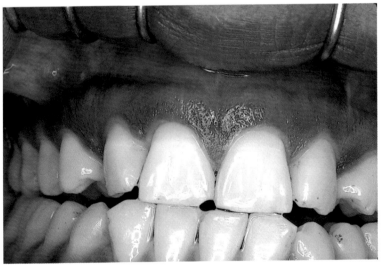

Fig. 220 Racial pigmentation of gum.

Index